Functional Informatics in Drug Discovery

Drug Discovery Series

Series Editor

Andrew Carmen

Johnson & Johnson PRD, LLC
San Diego, California, U.S.A.

Functional Informatics in Drug Discovery

Edited by
Sergey Ilyin

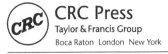

CRC Press
Taylor & Francis Group
Boca Raton London New York

CRC Press is an imprint of the
Taylor & Francis Group, an **informa** business

Published 2008 by CRC Press
Taylor & Francis Group
6000 Broken Sound Parkway NW, Suite 300
Boca Raton, FL 33487-2742

© 2008 by Taylor & Francis Group, LLC
CRC Press is an imprint of Taylor & Francis Group, an Informa business

First issued in paperback 2019

No claim to original U.S. Government works

ISBN-13: 978-0-367-45294-0 (pbk)
ISBN-13: 978-1-57444-466-7 (hbk)

Visit the Taylor & Francis Web site at
http://www.taylorandfrancis.com

and the CRC Press Web site at
http://www.crcpress.com

Library of Congress Cataloging-in-Publication Data

Functional informatics in drug discovery / edited by Sergey Ilyin.
    p. ; cm. -- (Drug discovery series ; 9)
  Includes bibliographical references and index.
  ISBN-13: 978-1-57444-466-7 (hardcover : alk. paper)
  ISBN-10: 1-57444-466-2 (hardcover : alk. paper)
  1. Bioinformatics. 2. Medical informatics. 3. Computational biology. 4.
Pharmaceutical technology--Data processing. I. Ilyin, Sergey. II. Series.
  [DNLM: 1. Computational Biology--methods. 2. Medical Informatics. 3.
Technology, Pharmaceutical--methods. QU 26.5 F979 2007]

QH324.2.F86 2007
615'.19--dc22
                           2007013029

Contents

Preface

The biopharmaceutical industry is facing tremendous and fascinating opportunities to improve its overall research and development and business efficiency by integrating various technologies and informational systems and by creating an intelligent interface between different systems and business segments. Currently there is no reference that has (a) looked into all of the different aspects of technology integration and information flow in the biopharmaceutical enterprise and (b) outlined the specifics and commonalities of technologies at different stages of development. An important and challenging aspect of this book is the in-depth analysis of emerging trends and future opportunities in integration and interfacing while maintaining a systematic or programmatic approach. This book comprises well-referenced updated chapters from leaders in the pharmaceutical industry, in academia, and in information technology. Each chapter reviews a particular area.

This book is intended for a heterogeneous audience, essentially anyone who seeks a greater understanding of the concepts and utilization of informatics. At the same time, sufficient detail and updated references are included so that scientists in any discipline, managers, and investors can benefit by better understanding these emerging trends and their applications.

Editor

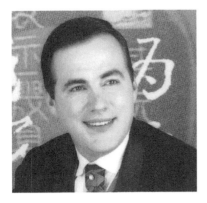

Sergey Ilyin graduated with distinction from the St. Petersburg State University in Russia with a combined B.Sc./M.Sc. degree in 1993. Following a fellowship at the Institute of Cytology of the Russian Academy of Sciences, he received an award from the Soros Foundation and accepted a full scholarship at the University of Delaware. Ilyin graduated from the University of Delaware with a Ph.D. degree in molecular biology/neuroimmunology under the mentorship of Professor Carlos R. Plata-Salaman, D.Sc., M.D., an expert in neurosciences with a focus in brain cytokine research. In this research, Ilyin described, for the first time, the integrative regulation of the brain interleukin-1 system under various pathophysiological conditions and in the induction and progression of anorexia in various models.

In 1999, Ilyin joined the Central Nervous System Research Team at the Johnson & Johnson Pharmaceutical Research Institute as a postdoctoral research fellow. Following this, Ilyin was promoted through positions of increasing scope and responsibility that included establishing novel targets, projects, screening technologies and participation in several key drug-discovery projects. Ilyin is currently a group leader of bioinformatics at the Spring House facility of the Johnson & Johnson Pharmaceutical Research and Development LLC.

He has pioneered bioinformatic approaches in drug discovery; has conducted or directed projects in the areas of CNS, analgesia, vascularity, metabolism, oncology, and enterology; and has developed new approaches for target identification and validation. His activities also include data management and integration as well as research on biological markers for disease, drug efficacy, and safety applications, including identification and analysis of mechanisms of action. His responsibilities were later extended to translational technologies and approaches, including noninvasive imaging.

Ilyin has extensive experience in collaborating with different functions and teams within the company as well as with external networks and academic groups. He has published more than 40 peer-reviewed articles and has editorial responsibilities for several journals and books.

Contributors

G. Mark Anderson
Centocor Research & Development, Inc.
Malvern, Pennsylvania

Greg M. Arndt
Johnson & Johnson Research Pty. Ltd.
Eveleigh, Australia

Douglas E. Brenneman
Johnson & Johnson Pharmaceutical
  Research and Development LLC
Spring House, Pennyslvania

Katherine R. Calvo
National Institutes of Health
Bethesda, Maryland

Andrew Carmen
Johnson & Johnson Pharmaceutical
  Research and Development LLC
San Diego, California

Qiming Chen
Centocor Research & Development, Inc.
Malvern, Pennsylvania

James M. Dixon
Johnson & Johnson Pharmaceutical
  Research and Development LLC
Spring House, Pennsylvania

Mark Flynn
Los Alamos National Laboratory
Los Alamos, New Mexico

Daniel Horowitz
Johnson & Johnson Pharmaceutical
  Research and Development LLC
Spring House, Pennsylvania

Bingren Hu
University of Miami School of
  Medicine
Miami, Florida

Sergey E. Ilyin
Johnson & Johnson Pharmaceutical
  Research and Development LLC
Spring House, Pennsylvania

Fredrik Kamme
Johnson & Johnson Pharmaceutical
  Research and Development LLC
San Diego, California

Garrett T. Kenyon
Los Alamos National Laboratory
Los Alamos, New Mexico

Lance A. Liotta
National Institutes of Health
Bethesda, Maryland

Changlu Liu
Johnson & Johnson Pharmaceutical
  Research and Development LLC
San Diego, California

Ewa Malatynska
Johnson & Johnson Pharmaceutical
  Research and Development LLC
Spring House, Pennsylvania

Bernd Meurers
David Geffen School of Medicine at
  UCLA
Los Angeles, California

Marian T. Nakada
Centocor Research & Development, Inc.
Malvern, Pennsylvania

Emanuel F. Petricoin
U.S. Food and Drug Administration
Bethesda, Maryland

Albert Pinhasov
Johnson & Johnson Pharmaceutical
  Research and Development LLC
Spring House, Pennsylvania

Carlos R. Plata-Salamán
Eli Lilly and Company
Indianapolis, Indiana

Daniel Rosenthal
Johnson & Johnson Pharmaceutical
  Research and Development LLC
Spring House, Pennsylvania

Bernard J. Scallon
Centocor Research & Development, Inc.
Malvern, Pennsylvania

Linda A. Snyder
Centocor Research & Development, Inc.
Malvern, Pennsylvania

Da-Thao Tran
Johnson & Johnson Pharmaceutical
  Research and Development LLC
San Diego, California

Anil H. Vaidya
Johnson & Johnson Pharmaceutical
  Research and Development LLC
Spring House, Pennsylvania

Ole Vesterqvist
Bristol-Myers Squibb Pharmaceutical
  Research Institute
Princeton, New Jersey

Hong Xin
Johnson & Johnson Pharmaceutical
  Research and Development LLC
Spring House, Pennsylvania

Li Yan
Centocor Research & Development, Inc.
Malvern, Pennsylvania

Jingxue Yu
Johnson & Johnson Pharmaceutical
  Research and Development LLC
San Diego, California

Jessica Zhu
Johnson & Johnson Pharmaceutical
  Research and Development LLC
San Diego, California

1 Intelligent Automation

James M. Dixon

CONTENTS

INTRODUCTION

Progress in science depends on the elucidation of new concepts as well as the development of better tools for carrying out scientific research. The tools for scientific research have traditionally included instruments for measurement and experimentation. The advent of computers has provided a powerful mechanism for use in scientific research. All applications of computers in science require the development of software. Software applications vary greatly from informatics to database management to intelligent automation. There even exists a multitude of examples that have merged automation and informatics to form what is known as functional informatics [1, 2]. No matter what the application, computers have become a great asset in expanding our scientific knowledge. Of particular note are the great strides in software advances in automation, specifically in laboratory automation. With the use of intelligent software, output can be obtained with little or no user intervention or data analysis. Processes that were previously bottlenecks have evolved to provide a wealth of data and useful information with the adaptation of intelligent automation. In this chapter we will visit reaction optimization and see how the expansion of its adaptation into the biological sciences can expedite data collection and analysis.

LABORATORY AUTOMATION

Over the past several decades there have been major developments in laboratory automation stemming from the emergence of systems capable of processing large numbers of samples in parallel [3–7]. Laboratory automation can range from simple automation, such as automated analysis instruments (i.e., Cell Lab Quanta® by Beckman Coulter, Inc.), to more-complex integrated systems, such as intelligent laboratory workstations (i.e., Biomek® 2000 Laboratory Automation Workstation by Beckman Coulter, Inc.).

The range of laboratory automation can be broken into two levels of user input: open-loop and closed-loop experimentation. In open-loop experimentation, an experiment or analysis is set up and run with no decisions made based on data from previous or ongoing experiments. More often than not, the experiment or analysis was only meant for serial evaluation, and decisions are not necessary. This allows for easy use of the instrument by scientists, but it restricts the utility of the instrument because few, if any, adaptive changes can be made to the experimentation. In contrast, in closed-loop experimentation, ongoing experiments are evaluated, and future experiments are pruned, altered, or spawned based on data from previous or ongoing experiments [8]. Current integrated systems are moving in the direction of closed-loop experimentation, which is flexible and configurable and would allow the automated system to be a walk-away device. In return, this approach offers the prospect of increased productivity while reducing scientist intervention.

One of the more beneficial aspects of integrated systems stems from powerful software that allows scheduling of experimentation. Multiple sets of experiments can be implemented in parallel through the use of a scheduler. A simple scheduler offsets the start time of intact experimental plans and interleaves (in a comblike manner) the individual commands of the respective plans. The resulting schedule consists of a set of experimental plans with offset start times; in this manner the total duration of the set of parallel experimental plans is generally compressed by up to tenfold compared with that for serial implementation [9]. More-complex schedulers exist that can order the experiments in a particular fashion, such as by user ranking or by shortest experiment duration first.

Automated experimentation instruments, created from the combination of computers with robotics, have been assembled for diverse applications ranging from high-throughput screening to library preparation to reaction optimization. Because there is a push toward more-intelligent automation, our efforts will concentrate on reaction optimization, which provides the most desirable benefits of intelligent design.

REACTION OPTIMIZATION

Diverse automation systems, ranging from batch reactors to multireactor workstations, have been constructed with the dominant application of performing reaction optimization. Reaction optimization, an unglamorous but integral component of scientific research, is essential for achieving high-yield products and for developing cost-effective and environmentally benign processes [10]. By definition, optimization implies the ability to perform experiments, to evaluate data, and to perform modified experiments in an effort to achieve improved results. Box and coworkers [11] were among the pioneers in reaction optimization. Their studies of evolutionary operation in industrial settings were developed over a half a century ago and still hold true today.

There is a large set of evolutionary approaches to perform reaction optimizations. The approaches can be broken into four algorithm categories: (a) parallel, (b) adaptive, (c) parallel adaptive, and (d) integrated. In the following sections, each type of optimization algorithm is described along with some examples of each type.

PARALLEL ALGORITHMS

One of the simplest conceptual approaches for reaction optimization, open-loop experimentation, involves the examination of all combinations of factors that affect a given reaction (i.e., a full factorial design). In the case of a search space defined by two factors, all points in a regular two-dimensional grid are examined. The resulting data can then be plotted to give a response surface. Response surfaces for reactions are very valuable to scientists, but generally are not widely available due to the extensive manual labor required to investigate a large number of experiments. One approach to minimize the extent of manual experimentation has been to employ partial factorial designs, which examine only part of the space and then employ statistical approaches to tease out interactions among factors. The methodology of statistically designed experiments is well developed, but it has made limited inroads among scientists.

Automated workstations provide the means to perform a vast number of experiments with minimal scientist intervention, which reduces the laborious task of performing tedious experiments and eliminates the need for statistical treatment. Thus, grid searches (factorial designs) can be a viable option for optimization. The fact that grid searches are performed with no decision-making features means that, upon completion of all experiments, the automation software can only decide whether and where an optimum value exists [12]. As previously mentioned, the duration of the experimentation is reduced dramatically by performing the experiments in parallel. What would have taken an exorbitant amount of time to obtain scientific data can be reduced to a manageable duration.

ADAPTIVE ALGORITHMS

Adaptive algorithms are the foundation of closed-loop experimentation. Algorithms that can make scientist-independent decisions have made great strides toward intelligent automation. One of the most commonly used adaptive algorithms is the simplex algorithm [13], which is a well-known method for hill-climbing optimization. Many modifications to the original simplex algorithm have been developed. Betteridge et al. [14] have devised a robust method, called the composite modified simplex (CMS), that combines the best features of various modified simplex methods [15].

A simplex is an n-dimensional polygon with $(n + 1)$ vertices, where n is the number of control variables for optimization and each vertex has n coordinates. The simplex is triangular in two-dimensional space, tetrahedral in three-dimensional space, and so forth. The optimization begins with a set of initial experiments whose number is equal to the number of control variables plus 1 ($n + 1$). According to the experimental results, the subsequent vertex is projected in a direction opposite from the worst vertex (Figure 1.1). The new simplex consists of one new point and n points from the previous simplex (i.e., discarding the worst point and replacing it with a new point). Consequently, despite the degree of the dimensional space, only a single

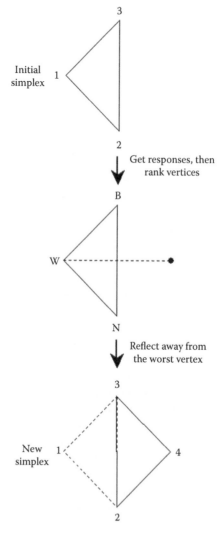

FIGURE 1.1 CMS movement. The basic simplex (i.e., CMS) moves in a two-dimensional search space. In an n-dimensional space, the simplex algorithm discards the one worst point in each simplex, maintains n points, and projects one new vertex with each move. The simplex algorithm requires serial implementation. (B: best response point; N: next best point; W: worst response point.)

experiment is proposed aside from the $(n + 1)$ points in the initial cycle. Repetitive measurements of the response and the reflection of simplices form the basis for the most elementary simplex algorithm. The CMS optimization is attractive because the calculations are straightforward, the search space is expandable to encompass multiple dimensions, and the method is robust in the presence of experimental noise [9].

PARALLEL ADAPTIVE ALGORITHMS

A fusion of parallel and adaptive algorithms is the culmination of efforts to create closed-loop experimentation. Parallel adaptive algorithms allow for wide searching of search spaces with convergent properties. A straightforward example of a parallel adaptive algorithm is a grid search that has evolutive properties to converge on an optimum response. A regular grid of points is examined in one cycle; then a second, more focused, grid is situated around the region of optimal response. A third even more tightly focused grid is then examined around the region of optimal response observed in the preceding cycle (Figure 1.2). In this manner, the entire search space is examined, the region of optimal response is identified, and an increasingly fine-grained search is implemented in the region of optimal response. This algorithm for experimentation affords both a coarse-grained response surface for the entire search space and a fine-grained evaluation in the region of greatest interest without requiring the entire search space to be examined with the same fine graining [16].

Another useful parallel adaptive algorithm is the multidirectional search (MDS) method. The MDS algorithm was created by Torczon to overcome the serial nature

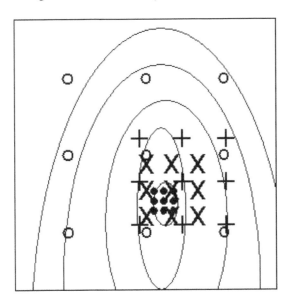

FIGURE 1.2 Successively focused grid searches. The first grid is cast broadly (O). The second grid (+) is centered around the point from the first grid that gave the highest point. A third grid (□) and fourth grid (•) are projected in a similar fashion. In this manner, the entire surface is examined in a coarse-grained fashion, and the optimal region is examined in a fine-grained fashion.

of the simplex method [17–20]. Torczon's work stemmed from considering how best to take advantage of multiple parallel processors in the computational evaluation of unconstrained optimization problems. The resulting MDS algorithm is also simplex-based, but differs in a fundamental way from the traditional simplex method. As previously stated, in a simplex algorithm, each move occurs by reflection away from the one worst point, creating a new simplex that contains one new point, regardless of search-space dimension. In each move, the one worst point is discarded, and the one new point of the new simplex is evaluated. In contrast, in the MDS method, each move occurs by reflection away from all but the one best point (Figure 1.3). The new simplex in n-dimensional space is composed of n new points and only the single best point from the previous simplex.

The MDS algorithm has a further distinction from that of a simplex movement. In addition to those points that are required to iterate simplex projections through the space (mandatory points), exploratory points can be evaluated in each cycle of MDS to the extent that resources are available to do so. The exploratory points are identified by the look-ahead projection of possible future simplexes. Examples of the range of exploratory points that can be examined for the initial cycle are shown in Figure 1.4. The number of experiments implemented per cycle depends on the dimension of the search space and the batch capacity of the workstation (which limits the number of exploratory experiments). Only one search space is investigated in a given course of experiments. The MDS method provides a means of evolutionary optimization via parallel experimentation. Thus, a simplex search projects only one new point per cycle, whereas MDS projects at least n new points per cycle [21].

Another approach to increase parallelism with simplex methods is to project multiple simplexes on a single search space. The simplex searches are independent in the direction of their movement but march in lockstep. A set of experiments of number equal to $m \times (n + 1)$ is generated as the initial trial, and m experiments are proposed for the subsequent cycle, where m is the number of independent simplex searches and n is the dimension of the search space. In a given search, the number of simplexes can be chosen by the user; the number generally can be determined by a set pattern to achieve an even distribution of initial simplexes, and the number increases with search-space dimension (Figure 1.5) [22, 23]. One of the greatest advantages of this method is that it minimizes an inherent flaw of simplex searches. With one simplex, convergence is possible on a local maximum/minimum. However, multiple simplexes have a much higher probability of converging on the global maximum/minimum because of the sheer number of converging simplexes.

INTEGRATED ALGORITHMS

Integrated algorithms combine the screening capabilities of parallel algorithms with the convergence properties of adaptive algorithms, but they do so in a unique way compared with parallel adaptive algorithms. There are many methods for integrating the different optimization algorithms. One particular example of interest is a technique that uses a two-tiered approach. The first tier employs a broad search to mark promising areas (breadth-first search). The second tier employs in-depth searches according to the results of the first-tier survey [24]. Figure 1.6 illustrates this

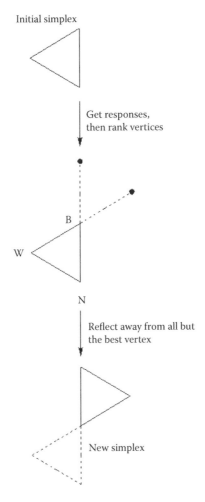

FIGURE 1.3 Basic MDS movement in a two-dimensional search space. In an *n*-dimensional space, the MDS algorithm discards *n* points in each simplex (all but the best), maintains the one best point, and projects *n* new vertices with each move. The MDS algorithm is amenable to parallel implementation. (B, N, and W are as defined in Figure 1.1.)

approach. This technique has several great advantages over normal methods of optimization: (1) less experimentation is performed because areas with a lower likelihood of having the optimum response are ignored, (2) focusing on the optimum response in the first tier allows the convergence of adaptive algorithms to remain fine grained, and (3) chemical and specimen samples are conserved because fewer resources are needed to perform an experiment.

Parallel, adaptive and integrated approaches take the best of both parallel and adaptive features, creating an amalgam of convergent and exploratory experimentation. This, in turn, provides a greater throughput and the possibility of walk-away experimentation compared with either parallel or adaptive experimentation individually.

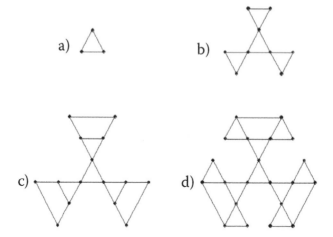

FIGURE 1.4 Projection of points in the MDS method. (a) Initial simplex. (b) The initial simplex and reflections from all vertices, with 6 exploratory points. (c) The initial simplex, reflections from all vertices, and expansions from all reflections, with 12 exploratory points. (d) The initial simplex, reflections from all vertices, expansions from all reflections, and reflections of all reflections, with 18 exploratory points.

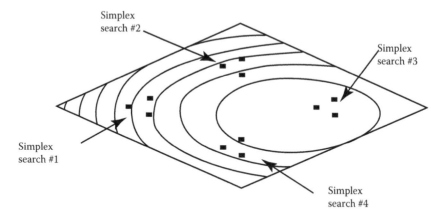

FIGURE 1.5 Multiple simplex projections. Distinct concurrent simplex searches in a single search space (two dimensional).

These combined approaches lend themselves nicely to automation and provide an avenue for future advances in reaction optimization.

OPTIMIZATION INTEGRATION

With recent advances in automation, there are ample opportunities to effectively integrate optimization techniques into the investigative environment of biological

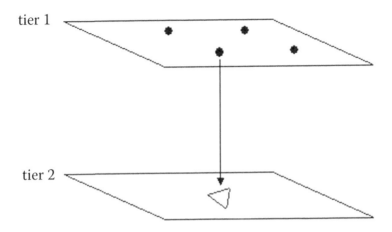

FIGURE 1.6 Two-tiered experimentation. A breadth-first survey identifies the appropriate starting point for a subsequent in-depth optimization with the CMS, MDS, or multiple simplex searches.

research laboratories. Many of the algorithms described previously for reaction optimization can be applied to other technologies. There are many genomic examples where this type of optimization can occur, such as polymerase chain reaction (PCR) primer design or other expression-profiling technologies. However, for simplicity, we will concentrate on a proteomic technology that is well established in a research environment and is very amenable to intelligent automation advancements: enzyme-linked immunosorbent assay (ELISA) development.

ELISA is a biochemical technique that is used to detect the presence of an antibody or an antigen in a sample. Two antibodies are used for this assay: one antibody is specific to the antigen, and the other, coupled to an enzyme, reacts to antigen–antibody complexes and causes a chromogenic or fluorogenic substrate to produce a detectable signal. ELISA assays are extremely useful tools both for determining serum antibody concentrations and for detecting the presence of antigen because they can be performed to evaluate either the presence of antigen or the presence of antibody in a sample [25].

Important diagnostic assays that have been developed, such as the tests for human immunodeficiency virus (HIV) or West Nile virus, have made ELISA assays commonplace in many biological laboratories. This, in turn, has made automation essential for quick diagnostic turnaround. There are many examples of automated ELISA workstations that can provide accurate and reliable results while allowing scientists to remain hands off.

AUTOMATED ELISA OPTIMIZATION WORKSTATION

Technology has accelerated ELISA experimentation to the point where ELISA "kits" or established protocols are all that are required for experimentation. Using developed kits and protocols, integration into automation is easily achieved. However, in a research laboratory, the use of high-throughput diagnostics is usually not enough. Many studies require optimization of the ELISA reagents and protocol before any useful information can be extracted from the experiment. Manual optimization can be tedious and time consuming, so an integration of optimization algorithms would greatly alleviate the laborious task of developing new assays. Simple offline optimization planning software is available to aid the scientist in setting up an optimization, but the scientist must manually prepare the ELISA in the planning software's scheme. Real-time optimization is relatively straightforward with previously automated processes. Thus integration of optimization algorithms would not be an immense undertaking, allowing for even greater throughput.

To develop an automated ELISA optimization, a workstation must be chosen that has considerably flexible components and a programming language that can create commands to accommodate real-time decision making (closed loop). As stated previously, the automation software used in the workstation should include features for composing experimental plans, managing resources (chemicals and containers), scheduling experiments, and evaluating data.

ELISA is a technology that displays a great number of optimization possibilities. In a general ELISA there are different types of buffers (i.e., coating, washing, and blocking), different chemicals/solutions for each type (i.e., albumin bovine serum in phosphate-buffered saline and nonfat dry milk for blocking buffers), and different concentrations of all chemicals and biologics involved. Each requires optimization for assay development to be effective. Using integrated or parallel adaptive algorithms, optimization can be set up to run on a single robotic workstation. Because the previously mentioned optimization algorithms can handle many parameters at once, each variable to be studied can be optimized in parallel on the workstation. To illustrate this point, let us look at the addition of the secondary antibody to an ELISA assay. This step is usually carried out using a predetermined dilution and type of antibody. For a new assay, this dilution and type are unknown and must be determined before the assay can be performed. In this case, an optimization can be carried out for each variable in the secondary optimization (i.e., secondary type and secondary concentration) using an algorithm such as MDS. Knowing that integrated algorithms and parallel adaptive algorithms can handle multiple dimensions or variables of an optimization, the entire secondary antibody step can be optimized in a single optimization run. This trend can continue for each step in the assay, so that the entire assay can be optimized in parallel on one workstation. The scheduler can organize the experiments so that there is no overlap in robotic use. The resulting intelligent automation will allow ELISA development to be very efficient and to be set up in a straightforward manner.

CONCLUSION

Advances in optimization software have opened new time-saving avenues that can enhance biological research. To be effective, the software must have intrinsic features of interest and yet be sufficiently "user friendly" to elicit the attention of experimental scientists. There are many solutions to intelligent automation analysis, but the utility of these solutions can be disputed based solely on their ease of use for a scientist. If this pitfall is avoided, the intelligent-automation solutions described in this chapter can have numerous applications and, if developed correctly, could advance progress in biological research, providing greater accuracy and time savings than ever before.

REFERENCES

1. Xin, H., et al., Throughput siRNA-based functional target validation. *J. Biomolecular Screening*, 2004. 9(4): 286–293.
2. Ilyin, S.E., et al., Functional informatics: convergence and integration of automation and bioinformatics. *Pharmacogenomics*, 2004. 5(6): 721–730.
3. Armstrong, J.W., A review of linear robotic systems for high throughput screening: new developments result in more flexibility and lower cost. *J. Assoc. Lab. Autom.*, 1999. 4(4): 28–29.
4. Gentsch, J., and O. Bruttger, High throughput screening at the nano scale. *J. Assoc. Lab. Autom.*, 2000. 5(3): 60–65.
5. Goodman, B.A., Managing the workflow of a high-throughput organic synthesis laboratory: a marriage of automation and information management technologies. *J. Assoc. Lab. Autom.*, 1999. 4(6): 48–52.
6. Hughes, I., Separating the wheat from the chaff: high throughput purification of chemical libraries. *J. Assoc. Lab. Autom.*, 2000. 5(2): 69–71.
7. Rose, D., and T. Lemmo, Challenges in implementing high-density formats for high throughput screening. *Lab. Autom. News*, 1997. 2(4): 12–19.
8. Du, H., et al., An automated microscale chemistry workstation capable of parallel, adaptive experimentation. *Chemom. Intell. Lab. Syst.*, 1999. 48: 181–203.
9. Corkan, L.A., and J.S. Lindsey, Experiment manager software for an automated chemistry workstation, including a scheduler for parallel experimentation. *Chemom. Intell. Lab. Syst.: Lab. Inf. Mgt.*, 1992. 17: 47–74.
10. Lindsey, J.S., Automated approaches toward reaction optimization. In *A Practical Guide to Combinatorial Chemistry*, A. Czarnik and S.H. DeWitt, Eds. American Chemical Society: Washington, DC, 1997, pp. 309–326.
11. Box, G.E.P., Evolutionary operation: a method of increasing industrial productivity. *App. Stat.*, 1957. 6: 81–101.
12. Kuo, P.Y., et al., A planning module for performing grid search, factorial design, and related combinatorial studies on an automated chemistry workstation. *Chemom. Intell. Lab. Syst.*, 1999. 48: 219–234.
13. Spendley, W., G.R. Hext, and F.R. Himsworth, Sequential application of simplex designs in optimization and evolutionary operation. *Technometrics*, 1962. 4: 441–461.
14. Betteridge, D., A.P. Wade, and A.G. Howard, Reflections on the modified simplex-I. *Talanta*, 1985. 32: 709–722.
15. Betteridge, D., A.P. Wade, and A.G. Howard, Reflections on the modified simplex-II. *Talanta*, 1985. 32: 723–734.
16. Dixon, J.M., et al., An experiment planner for performing successive focused grid searches with an automated chemistry workstation. *Chemom. Intell. Lab. Syst.*, 2002. 62: 115–128.
17. Dennis, J.E.J., and V.J. Torczon, Direct search methods on parallel machines. *SIAM J. Optimization*, 1991. 1: 448–474.

18. Torczon, V.J., Multi-directional search: a direct search algorithm for parallel machines. Ph.D. dissertation, *Department of Mathematical Sciences*. Rice University: Houston, TX, 1989.

19. Torczon, V.J., On the convergence of the multidirectional search algorithm. *SIAM J. Optimization*, 1991. 1: 123–145.

20. Torczon, V.J., On the convergence of pattern search algorithms. *SIAM J. Optimization*, 1997. 7: 1–25.

21. Du, H., S. Jindal, and J.S. Lindsey, Implementation of the multidirectional search algorithm on an automated chemistry workstation: a parallel yet adaptive approach for reaction optimization. *Chemom. Intell. Lab. Syst.*, 1999. 48: 235–256.

22. Matsumoto, T., H. Du, and J.S. Lindsey, A parallel simplex search method for use with an automated chemistry workstation. *Chemom. Intell. Lab. Syst.*, 2002. 62: 129–147.

23. Dixon, J.M. and J.S. Lindsey, An experiment planner for parallel multidirectional searches using an automated chemistry workstation. *J. Assoc. Lab. Autom.*, 2004. 9(6): 355–363.

24. Matsumoto, T., H. Du, and J.S. Lindsey, A two-tiered strategy for simplex and multidirectional optimization of reactions with an automated chemistry workstation. *Chemom. Intell. Lab. Syst.*, 2002. 62: 149–158.

25. Goldsby, R.A., et al., Enzyme-linked immunosorbent assay. In *Immunology*, 5th ed. New York: Freeman, 2003, pp. 148–150.

2 Neurally Inspired Algorithms as Computational Tools

Mark Flynn and Garrett T. Kenyon

CONTENTS

INTRODUCTION

One of the challenges facing the field of bioinformatics is the integration of large, multidimensional data sets. To understand biological processes at a systems level, data from multiple physiological components must be analyzed to uncover the dynamics governing their interactions. Currently, there are a multitude of databases covering mRNA and protein expression. To understand how changes in these domains reflect biological processes requires complex dynamic models to collate the many sets of data gathered to describe them. Models of related phenomena can then be compared to discover similarities and differences in their underlying dynamics and to understand changes over time and in response to perturbations. The development of such models should benefit from analytical tools for identifying and classifying expression motifs in bioinformatics data sets. However, such classification problems are fundamentally difficult, taxing even the most advanced techniques currently available.

The brain has evolved over millions of years into a highly efficient signal-processing and integration machine for classifying complex patterns. We propose that the same techniques employed by the brain to tackle particularly intractable problems, such as breaking a signal into discrete objects (signal **segmentation**), separating the signal from background noise (filtering), and the storage and recognition of complex patterns, can be utilized for the analysis of bioinformatics data sets. Advances in computing power and in our understanding of the brain have given us the ability to formulate usable computer models of neural functioning.

To form a representation of our sensory world, neural systems must interpret multiple, overlapping patterns of activity. For example, detectors of multiple features in the visual system, such as edges and corners, are activated at each point in our visual space. Likewise, each odor activates many olfactory neurons, and sounds trigger activity in a range of tone-sensitive neurons. Similar problems confront bioinformaticians. A disease process produces changes in many different genes/proteins. Multiple, overlapping patterns of gene expression coexist, reflecting the many processes in which each participates. A change in a single gene or protein rarely signifies a pathological state. A neuronal network-based bioinformatics tool could be used to segment the different patterns and to facilitate their classification as either physiological or pathophysiological.

Just as our brains create an internal representation of the sensory world, a neurally based computation tool would form a representation of multiple databases by processing the data and encoding local features as changes in the firing rates of simulated neurons. This tool then would group them into **cell assemblies** through **synchronous oscillations**, build up hierarchies of data assemblies, and combine them to form novel associations.

The question of how cell assemblies are formed addresses the core question of how the brain works. How does the brain form a sensory representation of the environment, store this representation, and make associations among its elements? Each sensory modality is initially processed separately in different areas of the cortex, and within each modality the stimuli are broken down further. For example, the visual world is processed into spatial and temporal components (the ventral and dorsal streams).[1] Somehow, these distributed representations of the sensory world must be reassembled to form coherent percepts, such as whole objects. Signal processing is a particularly intractable problem. The brain must be able to segment complex sensory stimuli and perform ill-posed, inverse mappings into appropriate categories. For example, our brains must be able to determine, from a flat projection on the retina, the identity and location in three-dimensional space of an object under widely different background and lighting conditions.

Our brains have a remarkable capacity for breaking down and reconstructing the world into coherent shapes that is unmatched by conventional computational techniques. Recent experiments have shed some light on the mechanisms responsible for this. One of these discoveries is that not only is information contained in the average spiking rate (the rate code), but it is also contained in the timing of the spikes (the temporal code).[2-9] The rate code (number of spikes in a given time period) indicates how strongly a neuron is activated. The temporal code (the relative timing of the spikes) is a property of a population of cells that can code for global properties of a stimulus,[10] for example whether the inputs to those cells are part of the same object or different objects.[11–13] In the visual system, cells that respond to contiguous stimuli will have a firing rate that synchronously oscillates,[11–13] while those that respond to different stimuli fire independently. Here we suggest that algorithms inspired by the brain can be used as tools for computer-based analysis of bioinformatics data sets and to test different theories about how the brain processes information. These two goals are complementary; better models of neural signal processing will produce better tools for computer-based data processing, while actual computer-based tools can help indicate where the current models can be improved.

This neuromimetic approach has many intrinsic advantages. Neural systems are naturally parallel, which produces advantages in processing speed and robustness to noise. Averaging over a population of neurons that are synchronously coupled allows for context-dependent noise filtering, as only those features that contribute to a given object need to be processed. Temporal coding can also be used to segment signals based on certain criteria, such as contiguity, smoothness, color, etc. The brain represents information in a hierarchical, distributed fashion, analogous to the distributed activation of multiple **biomarkers**. Because the brain has the ability to learn, it is not necessary to determine how best to represent the data ahead of time. The resulting model can be an emergent property of the data and the neural signal-processing system.

Synchronous oscillations have been found in many brain regions governing most aspects of neural functioning. These include the retina (Figure 2.1),[6,14,15] motor cortex,[16] hippocampus,[17] somatosensory cortex,[18,19] visual cortex, [4,10–13,20–30] and olfactory systems.[9,31–37]

Temporal coding is likely to be an important component of information processing in all neural systems. This chapter focuses on the role of temporal coding in three model systems that have been particularly well described, both experimentally and computationally — vision, olfaction, and hippocampal memory systems — focusing especially on those aspects potentially most useful for bioinformatics. Our goal is to suggest how lessons learned from these models can be used to build tools for processing bioinformatics data.

WHAT ARE SYNCHRONOUS OSCILLATIONS?

Synchronous oscillations are statistically significant quasi-periodic covariations in firing probability due to synaptic interactions rather than to changes in an external driving force, such as temporal modulation of the stimulus, or to purely intrinsic factors. Measurements of electroencephalograms (EEGs) have shown that there are rhythmic fluctuations in potential that can span large regions of the brain.[38] These oscillations are grouped into categories based on their frequency range, including theta (3–8 Hz), alpha (8–13 Hz), beta (15–30 Hz), and gamma (30–80 Hz) bands. Furthermore, measurements of the **local field potential** (LFP) inside the brain also exhibit these periodic oscillations.[16,26] Recordings using multielectrode arrays have shown synchronous oscillations in neural firing rates as well.[6,14,15,39] Firing-rate correlations can be quantified by examining the cross-correlation between two neurons, which indicates how likely it is that when one neuron spikes, the other one will spike at a given time before or after. Synchronous oscillations are revealed, for

a)

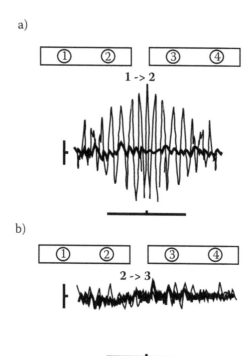

b)

FIGURE 2.1 Example of cross-correlograms (thin line) for (A) two retinal ganglion cell neurons responding to the same object whose firing is correlated and (B) for neurons responding to different objects whose firing is uncorrelated. The thick line is the shift predictor, which measures correlations that are time-locked to the stimulus (e.g., oscillations in the shift predictor might be directly due to stimulus coordination rather than network interactions). (Replotted from Kenyon, G. T., et al., *Vis. Neurosci.* 20, 465–480 [2003]. With permission.)

instance, when two neurons fire together more often than would occur solely due to chance and do so at quasi-periodic intervals.[40] Typically, the phases of synchronous oscillations recorded in the CNS drift randomly over time, so that correlations are rarely perfectly periodic and typically decline in amplitude over several cycles.

Synchronous oscillations have been proposed as a mechanism to dynamically bind neurons into cell assemblies.[41] These transient neuronal assemblies can define relationships between distributed neurons. Both multielectrode and EEG recordings have shown that neurons can synchronize over a wide range of spatial scales, both within and between cortical columns,[10,23] between cortical areas,[13] between hemispheres,[11,28] and between cortical and subcortical structures.[21,42]

Because synchronous oscillations are not solely the result of intrinsic cellular mechanisms, how do groups of neurons form dynamic cell assemblies? One proposed mechanism is that synchronous oscillations are due to delayed negative feedback between excitatory and inhibitory neurons.[43–46] The feedback inhibitory neurons act as "synchronizers" by entraining the excitatory neurons into oscillatory firing patterns. When the excitatory neurons fire action potentials, they excite the inhibitory feedback neurons, which project back in a broadly tuned fashion to inhibit the

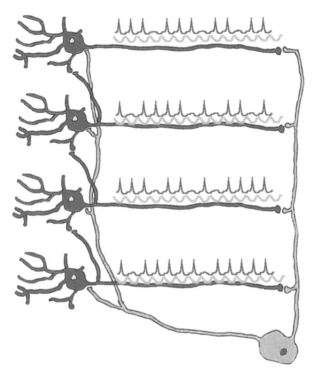

FIGURE 2.2 Feedback inhibition enforces synchronous oscillations by preventing the excitatory neurons from firing at the wrong time. The excitatory neurons (dark gray) activate the interneuron (light gray), which inhibits the excitatory neurons. While the excitatory neurons do not fire on every cycle, the feedback inhibition prevents them from firing out of phase.

excitatory neurons. This inhibition enforces a sort of refractory period, during which none of the neurons are likely to fire, and at the end of which neurons are more likely to fire due to rebound excitation. Such feedback circuitry may underlie the synchronous oscillations between retinal neurons (Figure 2.2).

Box 1

Recently elucidated plasticity rules suggest how such synchronously oscillatory circuits could emerge in a self-organizing fashion. Works from several labs[85–87] have demonstrated the effect that temporal structure has on the induction of plasticity. *In vitro* studies have shown that the temporal relationship in spiking between pre- and postsynaptic neurons affects synaptic efficacy. When the presynaptic neuron fires before the postsynaptic neuron, the synapse is potentiated; otherwise it is depressed. The temporal windows for LTP/LTD are asymmetric, with the window for potentiation much narrower than that for depression. So, only prepost pairings of less than 10 ms result in an increase in synaptic weight, and most other prepost intervals are depressing. Two neurons modulated by the

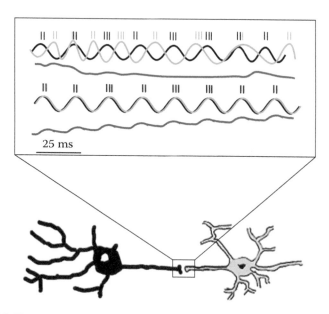

FIGURE 2.3 Phase relationship between pre- and postsynaptic neuron modulates synaptic gain. In this example, the presynaptic cell (in dark gray) is firing either in phase (bottom) or out of phase (top) with the postsynaptic cell (in light gray). The medium gray line under the sinusoids line is the synaptic gain. The regular pairings of presynaptic firing followed by postsynaptic firing produced by the synchronous oscillation results in a steady increase in synaptic strength, while the irregular firing of the asynchronous pair produces synaptic depression.

same underlying synchronous oscillation would produce the ideal phase relationship for spike-timing-dependent plasticity-mediated potentiation (Figure 2.3). Two decorrelated neurons, on the other hand, would fire spikes at random times relative to each other during the much longer window for depression and would become weakened.

It is possible that a common molecular mechanism underlies both coincidence detection and spike-timing-dependent plasticity, the NMDA (N-methyl-D-aspartate) receptor. NMDA requires two conditions for its activation, binding of glutamate and removal of Mg^{2+} blockade.[88] These two requirements impose a temporal order for NMDA activation. A presynaptic action potential causes the release of glutamate at an excitatory synapse. Binding of glutamate by the postsynaptic NMDA receptor opens the channel, but does not allow current to flow due to the Mg^{2+} ion blocking the channel. The arrival of a back-propagating action potential immediately after the binding of glutamate would depolarize the synaptic bouton, remove the Mg^{2+} ion, and allow the maximal entry of Ca^{2+} and Na^+. Using the same mechanisms, NMDA can act as a coincidence detector, or molecular phase detector, by enhancing synchronous PSPs in a nonlinear manner.

For neurons to form cell assemblies distributed across multiple brain regions, they must be able to reliably reproduce the temporal structure of their inputs. When a constant current is injected into a neuron, the temporal pattern of the resulting spike train is highly variable across many trials. However, when a realistic input current is injected into a neuron, the spike train is highly reproducible with a precision of less than 5 ms.[89] Neurons must also be able to detect input intervals of less than 5 ms as well.[90] Experiments have shown that differences of a few milliseconds can be detected. When an incoming EPSP is paired with a back-propagating action potential, the order in which they arrive at the synapse determines whether the gain of the synapse will be increased or decreased.[91]

Evidence from auditory and visual systems indicates that the brain makes use of this temporal precision. Single cell recordings show that spiking patterns in auditory cortex are reproducible with millisecond precision over multiple trials. In the visual system, temporal variations in retinal firing are reproduced in V1[14,21] and MT/V5.[92] This high degree of precision would be necessary to sustain these distributed assemblies of neurons across multiple synaptic relays.

ARGUMENTS FOR AND AGAINST SYNCHRONY

It has been argued that synchronous oscillations might not be important for neural coding.[47] One problem with encoding information in synchronous oscillations is that it can be difficult to distinguish true synchrony from chance correlations. A high level of stimulus-induced activity could create false synchrony simply due to the fact that the high number of spikes produces more coincident action potentials. Neurons would have to distinguish background synchrony from true synchrony for synchronous oscillations to encode useful information.

A property of neurons that can help to distinguish background from true synchrony is adaptation in the spiking threshold.[48,49] As the level of activity rises, the mean level of depolarization increases. The increase in threshold for spiking emphasizes rapid depolarization and increases the sensitivity to coincident inputs. This adaptive threshold mechanism narrows the window for coincidence and filters out temporally unpatterned input. This would decrease background synchrony and emphasize synchronous oscillations. Moreover, neurons can be sensitive to periodic input due to intrinsic or synaptic resonances at the appropriate frequency; in this case, aperiodic chance synchrony might be more easily distinguished from meaningful synchrony.

For synchronous oscillations to play a role in information processing, neurons must have mechanisms for discriminating between synchronous and asynchronous inputs. There have been several experiments that indicate that synchronously arriving postsynaptic potentials (PSPs) summate more effectively. Kenyon cells (KC) in the locust mushroom body have an intrinsic voltage-dependent mechanism for detecting coincident excitatory postsynaptic potentials (EPSPs).[35] When two different inputs to a cell arrived less than 12 ms from each other, a spike was evoked, but when the interval between inputs was greater than 12 ms or when the active conductances other than Na^+ and K^+ were blocked, no spike was produced.[35] In the hippocampal-slice preparation, correlated pre- and postsynaptic spikes that produced either long-term potentiation (LTP) or long-term depression (LTD) also changed how the postsynaptic cell integrated its input. Prepost pairings that produced LTP enhanced summation, while those that caused LTD decreased summation.[50]

Another issue is the theoretical problem with using synchrony to represent information across a group of neurons[51–53] as a population code. Averaging over a group of neurons can overcome some of the variability in individual neuronal firing. However, correlations between neurons could limit the advantage gained by averaging.[51–53] An illustrative analogy is a group of people independently estimating the weight of something. While the estimates may vary over a wide range, their mean will get closer to the true value as the number of individual estimates increases. However, when the estimates are not independent, for example in the stock market, where there are long-range correlations as everyone takes into account what everyone else thinks, there is a limit to the value of increasing the number of estimates. Synchrony in the responses would therefore limit the accuracy of the information encoded by a population of neurons in their average activity and would be a problem that the brain would need to overcome. However, information is not necessarily lost when the correlations themselves encode information.[54] Indeed, information lost due to correlations can be regained when the synchronous oscillations are stimulus dependent.[55]

EXAMPLES OF NEURONAL SYNCHRONY

Several neuronal systems make use of synchronous oscillations to process information, including, but not limited to, the visual, olfactory, and hippocampal memory systems.

VISION

One of the first brain regions where synchrony was detected was in the visual cortex,[4,21] followed by the lateral geniculate nucleus (LGN)[21] and the retina.[6,21] In all three areas, oscillations are dependent on properties of the stimulus, but are generated via synaptic interactions. Retinal ganglion cells oscillate synchronously to large spots, but not to small spots.[56] The oscillations can be mediated by inhibitory feedback via amacrine cells,[56,57] possibly augmented by the intrinsic properties of amacrine cells. Synchrony has not only been detected within brain areas, but also between them.[21] Neurons within the visual cortex oscillate most strongly to stimuli that produce the strongest firing response.[4]

Two problems faced by the visual system are image segmentation and feature binding. Information about each point in the visual space is carried along separate, parallel pathways. From the retina until at least the V2 cortex, each of these pathways is segregated into different channels based on color, motion, stereopsis, and shape. There are cells at each level of the visual processing system that respond preferentially to these different aspects of the visual world.

The problem of image segmentation relates to how the visual system determines which pixels belong to the same objects and which belong to different objects. One solution to this problem is to take advantage of the observation that neurons (for example, edge detectors in V1) responding to the same object oscillate synchronously, while neurons activated by different objects oscillate at random phase with respect to each other. A group of synchronously oscillating edge-detecting neurons would indicate that they are part of a single object boundary, or contour, and can therefore signal downstream visual areas that the responses from these neurons should be processed together. This has the additional benefit of improving the signal-to-noise ratio, since only objects above a certain size will produce synchronous oscillations.[56] A similar problem is encountered for the binding of the different aspects of visual objects (shape, motion, color, etc.). Synchronous oscillations could be used in the same fashion to bind these separate representations of the same object.

Groups of neurons across multiple spatial scales have been shown to oscillate synchronously, but what does such activity mean? One possibility is that synchronous oscillations could be useful for binding distributed representations of external stimuli (Figure 2.4). In addition, dynamically defined cell assemblies could act as a filter for downstream processing by signaling which neurons encode the information that is most relevant.[58] In particular, synchronous oscillations could be used as a feedback mechanism[3] to enhance elements that are responding to stimuli that require information outside of their receptive fields, for example a portion of a contour that is obscured. Another possibility is that synchrony could be used as a mechanism for linking cortical areas involved in a particular task into even larger cell assemblies. This would enhance the joint processing of stimuli related to the task while allowing unrelated activity to be ignored.

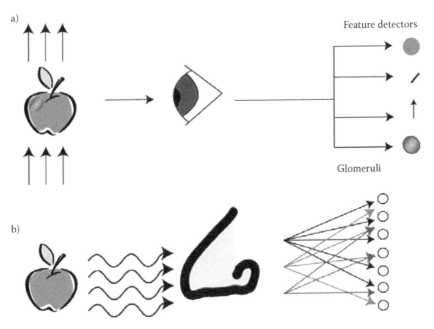

FIGURE 2.4 A given stimulus produces a response that is distributed across different processing channels within a sensory modality (e.g., color, motion, texture, and shape in the visual system) and across different modalities (e.g., sight and smell).

Binding of neurons into cell assemblies can be accomplished in two ways, either **binding by conjunction** or **dynamic binding**. Binding by conjunction uses a feed-forward, labeled-line strategy in which the firing rate of a downstream neuron is proportional to the presence of a particular conjunction of stimulus features, e.g., a corner-detecting neuron in the visual cortex that receives input from two edge-detector neurons and responds when both neurons increase their firing rates.

Dynamic binding is both feedforward and feedback. In this strategy, features are encoded by dynamic relationships among groups of neurons. Dynamic binding is implemented through transient neuronal assemblies. These assemblies consist of networks of broadly tuned elements that individually encode simple features that are bound into complex objects through synchronous oscillations. Thus, more-complex features are built from groups of synchronously oscillating neurons repre-senting simpler components. Instead of having a downstream cell that only responds to a particular combination of features at a particular scale, location, and orientation, dynamic combinations of complex objects are represented by simpler feature detec-tors that are oscillating synchronously. For example, two edge detectors might oscillate synchronously when responding to a single corner or closed contour. Thus, instead of needing a large number of downstream neurons — one for each unique conjunction of location, scale, and orientation of a given shape — a relatively small number of neurons is used to detect the presence of synchronously oscillating component features in a potentially viewpoint-independent manner. Binding by synchrony would also be useful for higher level visual processing. The higher up in the visual processing stream, the larger are the receptive fields and the more complex is the optimal stimulus for the neurons. More-complex objects could be represented by high-level neurons with broadly tuned rate-coded features bound together syn-chronously with neurons responding to lower-level features. Arbitrarily complex objects would consist of hierarchies of neuronal networks bound together by syn-chronous oscillations. In this way, a hierarchical network is built to represent more-complex features without requiring the combinatorially explosive number of neurons needed by a purely rate-coded network.

It is likely that both strategies are employed.[40] First, the neuronal responses are partially disambiguated by labeled-line code, as in retinotopic formation of edge detectors in the V1 cortex. Further separation of the population codes could be accom-plished by dynamic binding. Use of both strategies could be used to optimize both speed and flexibility. Frequently used or particularly relevant conjunctions could be represented by labeled-line, conjunction-specific neurons through long-term changes in neuronal connectivity. Many of these combinations could be represented implicitly via synchronous oscillations between the corresponding elements; new conjunctions could be represented by synchronous oscillations of the neurons responding to the component features.

OLFACTION

Another system where a functional role for synchrony has been demonstrated is the insect olfactory system. Indeed, the honeybee olfactory system has provided the most direct evidence that synchronous oscillations are critical for information processing. Selectively blocking synchronous oscillations impaired fine odor discrimination, but not of dissimilar odorants.[36] The problems of processing olfactory signals are similar to the demands on the visual system. Odors have distributed representations across receptors and must first be segmented into their individual components.

The role of synchronous oscillations has been investigated in several animal models of olfaction, including Drosophila, honeybee, locust, and zebrafish. While all have shown similar characteristics, the locust model is one of the best studied.[34] There are several types of receptors and receptor cells. Each receptor cell expresses exactly one receptor type. (The structure of the locust olfactory system is similar to what is shown in Figure 2.5; the locust equivalents of the mitral cells are the projection neurons, and the mushroom-body Kenyon cells are similar to piriform cortex.) Each receptor responds to several odors, and each odor activates several receptor types. All receptor cells expressing the same receptor type connect to the same glomeruli (not necessarily just one, but only a few), and the projection neurons (PNs) connect to one (or a few, depending whether in locust or other animals)

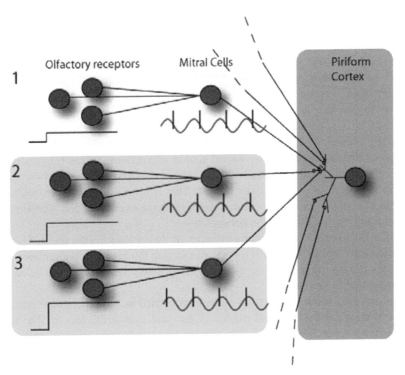

FIGURE 2.5 Activation of detectors is shown as a step-current injection, which is combined with oscillatory modulation to produce spikes at different times in the cycle. Mitral cell 3 receives the strongest input, and so it fires the earliest in the cycle. Neurons in the piriform cortex, if they have properties similar to those in the mushroom body, can then respond uniquely, depending on which mitral cells are firing and the temporal pattern of their input.

glomerulus (glomeruli). The antenna lobe (AL) consists of two types of cells, PNs and local neurons (LNs). The PNs connect to the intrinsic neurons of the mushroom body (MB), i.e., the Kenyon cells (KCs). There are many times more KCs than PNs. Each PN projects many KCs, and each KC receives input from multiple PNs.

The PNs respond to multiple odors in a unique odor-dependent fashion,[59] but the KCs respond to far fewer odors.[32] Activity in the AL forms a rough chemotropic map, with broad regions responding to similar odors and finer distinctions mapping to subregions of the AL.[60] However, since each PN responds to different odors, the identity of the PN is insufficient to signal the presence of a particular odor.

The locust olfactory system uses temporal patterning both to separate overlapping PN firing codes and to dilute (reduce the number of neurons necessary for) odor representation in the KCs.[61] The pattern of firing for similar odors in the AL, although unique, overlaps to a great extent. Slow temporal patterning over several seconds, with each neuron going through several epochs of increased and decreased firing, decorrelates the response to chemically related odors, decreasing their overlap. The combination of the identity of PNs firing and the temporal evolution of their firing rates helps to separate the overlapping PN rate code, thereby allowing the KCs to respond to a small subset of odors.[35]

As in the visual system, high-frequency synchronous oscillations play an important role in olfactory processing. KCs have several mechanisms that emphasize input from synchronously oscillating PNs. They have active conductances that shorten EPSPs so that only coincident input from PNs will summate. KCs only fire if most of their input PNs are firing, and then with only a few spikes. Also, background activity for the KCs is very close to zero, so any spiking signals the presence of its odor.

High-frequency LFP oscillations in the AL are a consequence of inhibitory local neuron → PN and local neuron → local neuron interactions. Spikes from individual PNs contributing to the oscillatory LFP are only locked to the oscillatory cycle during some epochs of the activity pattern. They drop in and out of the oscillation. Tuning characteristics of each neuron do not change over time, and sharpening of the odor representation is at the network level.[60]

Most KCs receive input from a minority of their PNs and stay silent. The large amount of divergence at the PN → KC connection dilutes the representation. Very few KCs fire during a stimulus, thus producing a very sparse code where an odor is represented by a few KCs.

Information about an olfactory stimulus is carried by both the spatial pattern of PN activation and the temporal pattern of fast- and slow-firing epochs. The spatial and temporal code from the AL is converted into a spatial code in the MB, which is optimal for linear classification.[62]

Temporal patterning in the olfactory system has a similar function in the visual system. Synchronous oscillations in the visual cortex serve as a mechanism for linking the activity of neurons responding to different aspects of the same stimulus. In the olfactory system, these oscillations help in disambiguating similar stimuli to create a more compact and efficient representation of a stimulus and to group neurons responding to different molecules that are a part of the same odor.

HIPPOCAMPUS

The hippocampus is an important structure for the encoding of memories.[63,64] Two types of memories are hippocampal dependent: episodic and semantic.[65] Episodic memory contains the important details of events, such as time, location, and the sensory environment. Semantic memory is the synthesis of episodic memories into a coherent framework in which (a) the details of an experience are fused into a generalized representation of similar experiences and (b) the elements of an episode are linked to similar elements in different experiences. The formation of semantic memory involves the linking of the different brain areas that mediate sensory perception, the conjunctions of events and places for a particular experience, and the common elements of many experiences. Another common aspect of experimentally observed hippocampal functioning is what are called "place cells." These are neurons that fire whenever the subject is at a particular location.[66] Other neurons are path specific; they fire at a particular location, but depend on where the subject started or where the subject will go.[67]

As in the other systems presented previously, the hippocampus uses both rate and temporal codes. An increase in firing rate is seen for both place cells and path-specific cells.[67] Two different oscillatory frequency bands are prominent in the hippocampus: the theta (5–10 Hz) and gamma (20–80 Hz) bands.[68] Theta oscillations have been linked to the encoding and retrieval of memory,[69–72] and gamma oscillations are responsible for the coordination of cortical regions that process the sensory and cognitive components that make up a memory. Gamma oscillations are well suited for this, as they can mediate long-range interactions. They are also transient in nature and thus can be rapidly coupled and decoupled to form new memories.

A model for short-term memory based on synchronous oscillations has been proposed (Figure 2.6).[73] Simulated neurons were given two different inputs: one with the information to be stored and the other a low-frequency oscillatory input. When the informational input is given during the oscillation, it produces an afterdepolarization (ADP) that causes it to continue to fire on subsequent cycles. In this model, memories are formed by these transient increases in membrane excitability and are refreshed by network oscillations. The time course of the ADP leads to an ordering of the groups of neurons, storing each memory into several nonoverlapping cell assemblies that fire synchronously during a particular subcycle. The synchronous firing of the neurons dissipates over time and thus requires the two oscillations to refresh synchrony.

The experimental finding that we can hold 7 ± 2 chunks of information in our short-term memory at one time has become well known.[74] Each of the individual elements contained in our short-term memory is stored within the gamma subcycle of the overall theta rhythm. So, with the 40-Hz gamma oscillations and 6-Hz theta oscillations, they can hold about seven elements at a time. As new elements come in, they would enter at the beginning of the theta cycle and displace those at the last subcycle of the gamma queue. The position within the gamma queue defines the temporal relationships among the elements in memory, and so the position would put events into their proper temporal order.

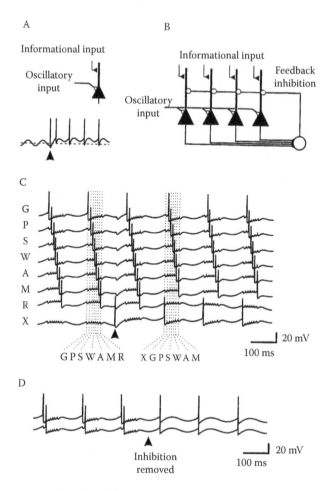

FIGURE 2.6 Proposed model of short-term memory. (A) Modulation of the excitability of neurons by a theta oscillation allows a group of neurons to fire during the same cycle. (B) Feedback inhibition produces a gamma oscillation. (C) The network can maintain multiple items in short-term memory, with each subcycle of the gamma oscillation containing a different memory. (D) The feedback inhibition is necessary for the gamma oscillation and for maintaining the relative phase information for the different elements in memory. (From Lisman, J. E., and Idiart, M. A. *Science* 267, 1512–1515 [1995]. With permission.)

Current Approaches

The first neurally based technique, artificial neural network (ANN), has been studied for many years and has recently been used for bioinformatics problems.[93] A neural network consists of one or more connected layers of neuronlike nodes. Each neuron nonlinearly sums up its inputs, and if these exceed the neuron's threshold, the neuron sends a signal to its outputs. The strengths or weights of the connections are set during a training phase, depending on the particular learning rule used and the set of inputs used for training. They have been used in many applications involving multifactorial classification and multivariate nonlinear regression, which would make them useful tools for analyzing complex data sets.[94]

ANNs are particularly suited for image analysis and pattern recognition.[93] One important task involving pattern recognition is predicting the structure of a protein from its amino acid sequence. ANNs have been used to find the secondary structure of proteins[95] and to determine the individual amino acid solvent accessibility.[96] Proteins with known structures are used as the training set for the neural network. This training modifies the connection weights between the nodes so that the neural network builds a model of the relationship between amino acid sequences and secondary structure or solvent accessibility. The neural network can then be used to search for similar patterns of amino acids to predict the structure of unknown proteins.

A neuromimetic approach, which uses more-realistic, spiking neurons, should in principle be more effective at pattern recognition. A spiking neuronal network has an additional channel of information that is unavailable to a non-spiking neural network: the temporal structure of the spike train. This extra channel can be used to encode information that is unavailable to an individual node, for example to the global context in which the unit is embedded.

APPLICATIONS OF TEMPORAL CODING IN SIGNAL PROCESSING

Processing strategies employed by natural neuronal systems could have potential benefit for signal processing and integration. The system with the most obvious applications is the visual system. Current techniques cannot match the speed and robustness of human vision. One obvious application is using a neurally based algorithm for segmentation of data from imaging techniques such as functional magnetic resonance imaging (fMRI), *in situ* hybridization, and confocal microscopy. This would involve converting an image into a matrix of current injections proportional to each pixel's gray-scale value and using that as input into a computational model of the visual system.

Earlier work with a model of the retina[56,57] showed that synchronous oscillations have characteristics that make computational vision models useful tools for image processing (Figure 2.7). The power of synchronous oscillations is proportional to the size of the stimulus, which makes them useful for noise filtering and for discriminating large-vs.-small objects as well as rapid segmentation. Depending upon the desired feature size, the sensitivity to noise can be set by the user. One of the key insights from this spiking-neuron model is that delayed inhibition is necessary for synchronous oscillations. So, by adjusting the gain and the time constant of the inhibition, one can control the power of the oscillations and thus the degree of filtering. The retinal model emphasizes adjacent pixels with roughly equivalent contrast by grouping them into synchronous blobs. Performance should improve for a model based on cortical V1 neurons.

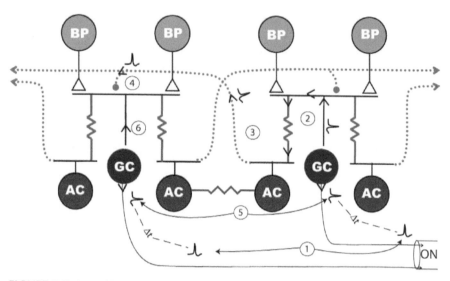

FIGURE 2.7 An oscillatory feedback loop in a retinal model. 1) Stimulation of the ganglion cells by the bipolar cells produces action potentials that propagate down the optic nerve. 2) Simultaneously, action potentials back-propagate through the dendrites of the ganglion cells, across gap junctions, and activate amacrine cells. 3) The spiking amacrine cells send action potentials along their axons to 4) inhibit the adjacent ganglion cells. 5) This delays spiking in the ganglion cells until the release of amacrine cell inhibition and so produces an interval with no spikes (t). 6) The feedback loop is completed by back-propagating spikes from the ganglion on the left traveling back to the ganglion cell on the right. Arrowheads indicate direction of action potentials. bipolar cells (BP), amacrine cells (AC), retinal ganglion cells (GC), and optic nerve (ON). Adapted from Stephens et al. (2006). (From Stephens, G. J., Neuenschwander, S., George, J. S., Singer, W. & Kenyon, G. T. See globally, spike locally: oscillations in a retinal model encode large visual features. *Biol Cybern* **95**, 327-348 (2006).)

A computational model of oriented edge detectors would allow more-complex segmentation than the retinal model. There is also the potential to combine all of the different types of cortical detectors into a single network that can segment based on color, texture, motion, and binocular disparity. Figure 2.8 shows a diagram of a model of V1 edge detectors developed for this purpose. They are equivalent to simple cells as described by Hubel and Wiesel.[77,78] These simple cells are modeled after pyramidal neurons in layer 4C and receive their primary input from the LGN. To simplify the model, input to the network is implemented as current injections. Oriented receptive fields are formed by retinotopic projections to V1 along the orientation preference (i.e., a vertical edge detector would receive input from a vertical line of input cells). The stimulus later also provides input to three groups of inhibitory interneurons: oriented feedforward, nonoriented feedforward, and inhibitory feedback. The interneurons inhibit the pyramidal cells and also form a mutually inhibitory loop. The feedforward interneurons sharpen the orientation tuning of the pyramidal neurons, and the feedback interneurons provide the slow inhibition to pyramidal cells necessary for oscillations. The internal feedback loop increases the dynamic range of the inhibitory interneurons and thus helps to keep the orientation

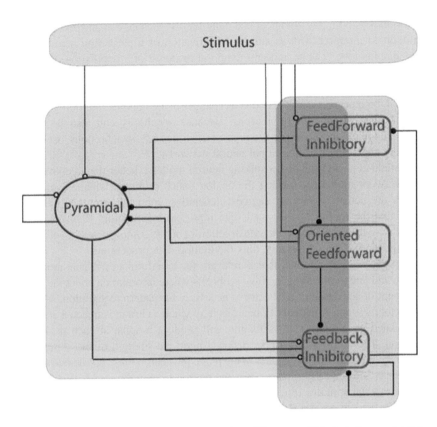

FIGURE 2.8 Diagram of network model based on V1 cortex. Filled circles are inhibitory synapses and hollow circles are excitatory synapses. Receptive fields for the pyramidal neurons and oriented feedforward inhibitory neurons are formed according to the model of Hubel and Wiesel.[77,78]

tuning insensitive to changes in contrast. Finally, the pyramidal neurons mutually excite each other. This excitation is selective and is designed to enhance the interactions between neurons that would fall along a smooth curve.[79] The connections between two neurons whose receptive fields (both orientational and positional in visual space) are tangent to the same circle have the maximal synaptic weight.[79]

To get smooth contours to oscillate synchronously, two elements are necessary: mutual excitation of neurons along the contour (cocircularity) and slow feedback inhibition. Slow feedback inhibition prevents a pyramidal cell from firing unless the other neurons are also firing. Cocircular connections help to ensure that most of the neurons along the contour fire at the peak of the cycle and extend the oscillations along the curve. Synchronous oscillations are used as a tag for all of the pixels in an image that belong to the same object. Each object in an image would have a different tag to assist in further processing.

The problems solved by the olfactory system are analogous to the problem of analyzing biomarker data to determine the efficacy of a drug. Each involves the analysis of output from multiple detectors. Because multiple processes modulate each biomarker, both physiological and pathological, a change in any one biomarker is difficult to interpret. This is similar to activation of a projection neuron in the locust antenna lobe. The spatial and temporal response of a population of neurons is necessary to identify an odor. A potentially powerful bioinformatics tool could be based on the olfactory system, in which both the presence and the magnitude of changes in biomarkers would be coded as changes in the number and timing of action potentials in a population of neurons. Because synchrony can also be used to dynamically bind the different features of a stimulus,[80] synchronous oscillations extend the capabilities of traditional neural networks.[81,82]

Hopfield et al. showed that a spiking neuron model is better than a conventional neural network model for solving the analog match problem, where several input channels are active to varying degrees, depending upon the stimulus.[83] Both the number and the timing of the spikes can represent information. Realistic spiking neurons may therefore allow the construction of more-complex models of data by encoding information temporally, thus facilitating data processing.

Hopfield presents a model that is relevant for bioinformatics.[84] This model uses both rate and temporal coding to solve problems where information about the identity and amount of activation of a detector is necessary for pattern recognition, such as in the olfactory system. A network of neurons into which a current is injected and which is modulated by a sinusoidal oscillation will produce a spike at each peak of the oscillation. The timing of the spike depends upon the strength of the stimulus: the stronger the input current, the earlier in the phase the neuron fires. The degree to which a detector is activated determines when the neuron fires in the cycle. Thus the characteristics of the stimulus (the ratios of the different components) are encoded as a temporal pattern of activity in the principal cells of the olfactory bulb. This temporal pattern can be decoded in the cortex by neurons sensitive to the timing of their inputs.

One problem with analyzing biomarkers is the need to compare changes in a scale-invariant manner. A disease process or pharmacologic response will produce a pattern of changes in a set of biomarkers (Figure 2.9). The ratio of these changes and the different scales at which they are measured are important factors in recognizing these patterns. This is a problem the olfactory system has solved. Odors are complex mixtures of airborne molecules where the minor components can be an important part of the odor.

Another possibility is to use an olfactory network-based model as a tool for molecular detection. The first step would involve separating a complex mixture into its component molecules using either gas or liquid chromatography. Each molecule could then be analyzed using a mass spectrometer (to get its molecular weight) and an infrared spectrometer (to determine the molecule's functional groups). The output from these devices could then be converted into a pattern of input currents for the olfactory network. Finally, these patterns could be decorrelated from similar molecules with overlapping PN patterns, and the representation could be diluted by the divergent PN projections to the Kenyon cells. A broad chemotropic map in the model antenna lobe could be based on a combination of molecular weight, hydrophobicity, and isoelectric point. Mapping within each subregion could be based on the molecule's functional groups.

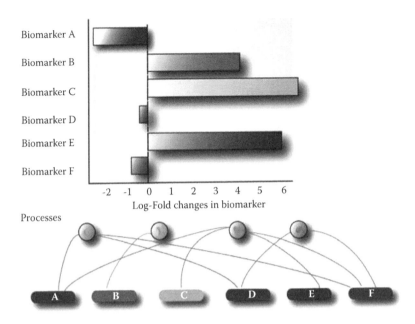

FIGURE 2.9 (A) Changes in levels of biomarkers after pathologic or pharmacologic perturbation. (B) Different processes could be modulating those biomarkers, making it difficult to interpret any changes.

A system of tools could be constructed from multiple neuronal networks to discover complex, multidimensional associations (Figure 2.10). For example, the effects of a series of drugs can be characterized by a series of *in situ* hybridization images. A visual-cortex-based tool could analyze these images, and an olfactory network could store the drugs. Then, correlations between the *in situ* images and the molecular profile of the drug could be systematically explored.

Higher Cognitive Functions

Synchronous oscillations have also been proposed to be the foundation of other complex phenomena, such as decision making, attention, and consciousness.[38] Attentional mechanisms bias processing toward the brain regions necessary for a task. Global synchronous oscillations make up the "dynamic core" of conscious behavior, while local oscillations involved in lower-level functions such as sensory processing would be subconscious (Figure 2.11). Cognition requires the large-scale coordination of multiple neuronal networks. Deficits in synchronous activity have been linked to pathologies involving large-scale neuronal network coordination, including schizophrenia[75] and autism.[76]

Our brains naturally tend to break complex objects into simpler components, just as we build up complicated concepts from simpler ideas. One conceivable

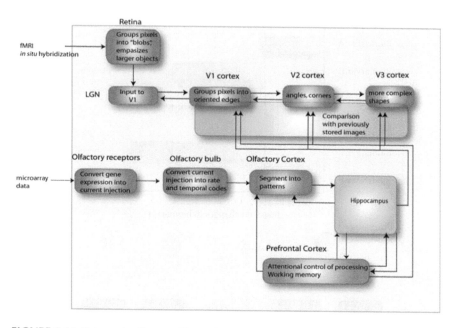

FIGURE 2.10 Schematic diagram illustrating a potential tool for constructing a neuronal network-based data model. Data are encoded through either visual or olfactory networks, depending on the characteristics of the data. Associations between elements of the data are formed by the hippocampus. The user could define important types of associations that could be enhanced by the prefrontal cortex network by increasing the power of oscillations in the target brain regions.

mechanism for how our brains accomplish this is to dynamically bind the neural circuits (themselves bound by synchronous oscillations) encompassing the simple components together via gamma-band synchronous oscillations. Indeed, even novel ideas could be generated by the transient confluence of previously unconnected neural assemblies. The components must already be present if the mind is to make the linkage.

As neuronal models that instantiate these principles become more complex, the more such models enter the realm of artificial intelligence (AI).[97] Indeed, this may be a prerequisite for truly powerful bioinformatics tools. This approach to AI might have some substantial advantages over conventional AI techniques,[98] which include expert systems, agent-based networks, neural networks, and semantic networks. These coarse-grained, high-level approaches require built-in representation of the problems they solve and have limited flexibility to handle unforeseen conjunctions of data. A bottom-up model of cognition allows the system to determine its own representation of the problem and provides the flexibility to link the very different types of data required by different cognitive tasks.

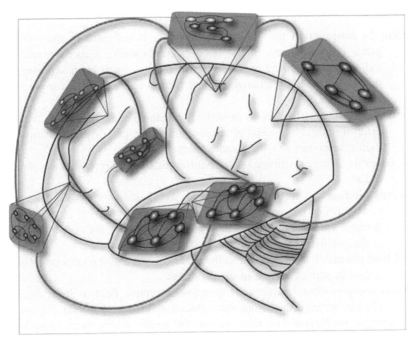

FIGURE 2.11 Synchronous oscillations link activity across brain regions to form cell assemblies.

CONCLUSION

Our brains formulate models of how the world works by integrating information about our visual, olfactory, tactile, and auditory environments into an existing body of knowledge. Algorithms based on the neural processes that perform these tasks should, in principle, be a useful strategy for making sense of the vast amounts of data generated in the fields of genomics, proteomics, metabonomics, and metabolomics. Neuronal networks that incorporate temporal coding have many useful characteristics. Because synchronous oscillations in the visual system scale with the size of the object, they can act as a context-dependent noise filter. The presence of a feature is indicated by identifying the neurons that respond to that feature, with the firing rate being proportional to the contrast or local signal strength. Contextual factors, such as the presence of cocircular elements, are encoded by the timing of the neuron's spikes. A network that includes the visual, olfactory, and hippocampal memory systems could encode a set of biomarkers and discern novel associations between different sets of markers. One of the key lessons learned from the brain that could be useful for bioinformatics is the possibility of binding data from these different sources to gain insight into the fundamental questions of biology.

GLOSSARY

binding by conjunction the presence of a feature is indicated by the convergence of components of the feature. For example, a corner could be indicated by the firing of a neuron that receives input from two neurons that are activated by a horizontal and vertical line at a particular place in visual space.

biomarker a characteristic that is objectively measured and evaluated as an indicator of normal biological processes, pathogenic processes, or pharmacological responses to a therapeutic intervention.

cell assembly a large distributed set of neurons that jointly represent a common object.

dynamic binding the presence of a feature is indicated by the dynamic interactions between neurons rather than through convergence of inputs onto a detector neuron. Each neuron has a piece of the puzzle, and only by looking at the population can the whole picture be seen.

local field potential averaged extracellular activity for a group of neurons consisting mostly of current in the dendrites.

sensory segmentation linking activity across receptive field to form distinct objects, distinguished from other objects and the background.

synchronous oscillation two neurons that fire action potentials in phase with each other.

ACKNOWLEDGMENTS

I thank Thomas Nowotny for his valuable comments on the manuscript. This work is supported by the DCI Postdoctoral Fellowship Program.

REFERENCES

1. Goodale, M. A., and Milner, A. D. Separate visual pathways for perception and action. *Trends Neurosci.* 15, 20–25 (1992).
2. Beaudot, W. H. Role of onset asynchrony in contour integration. *Vision Res.* 42, 1–9 (2002).
3. Engel, A. K., Fries, P., and Singer, W. Dynamic predictions: oscillations and synchrony in top-down processing. *Nat. Rev. Neurosci.* 2, 704–716 (2001).
4. Gray, C. M., and Singer, W. Stimulus-specific neuronal oscillations in orientation columns of cat visual cortex. *Proc. Natl. Acad. Sci. USA* 86, 1698–1702 (1989).
5. Lamme, V. A., Super, H., Landman, R., Roelfsema, P. R., and Spekreijse, H. The role of primary visual cortex (V1) in visual awareness. *Vision Res.* 40, 1507–1521 (2000).
6. Neuenschwander, S., Castelo-Branco, M., and Singer, W. Synchronous oscillations in the cat retina. *Vision Res.* 39, 2485–2497 (1999).
7. Nicolelis, M. A., Baccala, L. A., Lin, R. C., and Chapin, J. K. Sensorimotor encoding by synchronous neural ensemble activity at multiple levels of the somatosensory system. *Science* 268, 1353–1358 (1995).

8. Sauve, K. Gamma-band synchronous oscillations: recent evidence regarding their functional significance. *Conscious Cogn.* 8, 213–224 (1999).

9. Teyke, T., and Gelperin, A. Olfactory oscillations augment odor discrimination not odor identification by Limax CNS. *Neuroreport* 10, 1061–1068 (1999).

10. Gray, C. M., Konig, P., Engel, A. K., and Singer, W. Oscillatory responses in cat visual cortex exhibit inter-columnar synchronization which reflects global stimulus properties. *Nature* 338, 334–337 (1989).

11. Engel, A. K., Konig, P., Kreiter, A. K., and Singer, W. Interhemispheric synchronization of oscillatory neuronal responses in cat visual cortex. *Science* 252, 1177–1179 (1991).

12. Engel, A. K., Konig, P., and Singer, W. Direct physiological evidence for scene segmentation by temporal coding. *Proc. Natl. Acad. Sci. USA* 88, 9136–9140 (1991).

13. Engel, A. K., Kreiter, A. K., Konig, P., and Singer, W. Synchronization of oscillatory neuronal responses between striate and extrastriate visual cortical areas of the cat. *Proc. Natl. Acad. Sci. USA* 88, 6048–6052 (1991).

14. Neuenschwander, S., and Singer, W. Long-range synchronization of oscillatory light responses in the cat retina and lateral geniculate nucleus. *Nature* 379, 728–732 (1996).

15. Ishikane, H., Kawana, A., and Tachibana, M. Short- and long-range synchronous activities in dimming detectors of the frog retina. *Vis. Neurosci.* 16, 1001–1014 (1999).

16. Baker, S. N., Kilner, J. M., Pinches, E. M., and Lemon, R. N. The role of synchrony and oscillations in the motor output. *Exp. Brain Res.* 128, 109–117 (1999).

17. Bragin, A., et al. Gamma (40–100 Hz) oscillation in the hippocampus of the behaving rat. *J. Neurosci.* 15, 47–60 (1995).

18. Murthy, V. N., and Fetz, E. E. Coherent 25- to 35-Hz oscillations in the sensorimotor cortex of awake behaving monkeys. *Proc. Natl. Acad. Sci. USA* 89, 5670–5674 (1992).

19. Fetz, E. E., Chen, D., Murthy, V. N., and Matsumura, M. Synaptic interactions mediating synchrony and oscillations in primate sensorimotor cortex. *J. Physiol. Paris* 94, 323–331 (2000).

20. Brosch, M., Bauer, R., and Eckhorn, R. Synchronous high-frequency oscillations in cat area 18. *Eur. J. Neurosci.* 7, 86–95 (1995).

21. Castelo-Branco, M., Neuenschwander, S., and Singer, W. Synchronization of visual responses between the cortex, lateral geniculate nucleus, and retina in the anesthetized cat. *J. Neurosci.* 18, 6395–6410 (1998).

22. Deppisch, J., Pawelzik, K., and Geisel, T. Uncovering the synchronization dynamics from correlated neuronal activity quantifies assembly formation. *Biol. Cybern.* 71, 387–399 (1994).

23. Engel, A. K., Konig, P., Gray, C. M., and Singer, W. Stimulus-dependent neuronal oscillations in cat visual cortex: inter-columnar interaction as determined by cross-correlation analysis. *Eur. J. Neurosci.* 2, 588–606 (1990).

24. Ernst, U., Pawelzik, K., Tsodyks, M., and Sejnowski, T. J. Relation between retino-topical and orientation maps in visual cortex. *Neural Comput.* 11, 375–379 (1999).

25. Gray, C. M., Engel, A. K., Konig, P., and Singer, W. Stimulus-dependent neuronal oscillations in cat visual cortex: receptive field properties and feature dependence. *Eur. J. Neurosci.* 2, 607–619 (1990).

26. Gray, C. M., Engel, A. K., Konig, P., and Singer, W. Synchronization of oscillatory neuronal responses in cat striate cortex: temporal properties. *Vis. Neurosci.* 8, 337–347 (1992).

27. Gray, C. M., and Viana Di Prisco, G. Stimulus-dependent neuronal oscillations and local synchronization in striate cortex of the alert cat. *J. Neurosci.* 17, 3239–3253 (1997).

28. Konig, P., Engel, A. K., and Singer, W. Relation between oscillatory activity and long-range synchronization in cat visual cortex. *Proc. Natl. Acad. Sci. USA* 92, 290–294 (1995).

29. Kreiter, A. K., and Singer, W. Stimulus-dependent synchronization of neuronal responses in the visual cortex of the awake macaque monkey. *J. Neurosci.* 16, 2381–2396 (1996).

30. Wachtler, T., Sejnowski, T. J., and Albright, T. D. Representation of color stimuli in awake macaque primary visual cortex. *Neuron* 37, 681–691 (2003).

31. Hopfield, J. J. Olfactory computation and object perception. *Proc. Natl. Acad. Sci. USA* 88, 6462–6466 (1991).

32. Laurent, G., and Naraghi, M. Odorant-induced oscillations in the mushroom bodies of the locust. *J. Neurosci.* 14, 2993–3004 (1994).

33. Nusser, Z., Kay, L. M., Laurent, G., Homanics, G. E., and Mody, I. Disruption of GABA(A) receptors on GABAergic interneurons leads to increased oscillatory power in the olfactory bulb network. *J. Neurophysiol.* 86, 2823–2833 (2001).

34. Perez-Orive, J., et al. Oscillations and sparsening of odor representations in the mushroom body. *Science* 297, 359–365 (2002).

35. Perez-Orive, J., Bazhenov, M., and Laurent, G. Intrinsic and circuit properties favor coincidence detection for decoding oscillatory input. *J. Neurosci.* 24, 6037–6047 (2004).

36. Stopfer, M., Bhagavan, S., Smith, B. H., and Laurent, G. Impaired odour discrimination on desynchronization of odour-encoding neural assemblies. *Nature* 390, 70–74 (1997).

37. Wehr, M., and Laurent, G. Relationship between afferent and central temporal patterns in the locust olfactory system. *J. Neurosci.* 19, 381–390 (1999).

38. Varela, F., Lachaux, J. P., Rodriguez, E., and Martinerie, J. The brainweb: phase synchronization and large-scale integration. *Nat. Rev. Neurosci.* 2, 229–239 (2001). (A review of the role of synchronous oscillations in the emergence of high-level cognitive functions.)

39. Roelfsema, P. R., Konig, P., Engel, A. K., Sireteanu, R., and Singer, W. Reduced synchronization in the visual cortex of cats with strabismic amblyopia. *Eur. J. Neurosci.* 6, 1645–1655 (1994).

40. Singer, W. Neuronal synchrony: a versatile code for the definition of relations? *Neuron* 24, 49–65, 111–125 (1999). (An excellent review of the role of synchrony in sensory processing.)

41. Singer, W., et al. Formation of cortical cell assemblies. *Cold Spring Harb. Symp. Quant. Biol.* 55, 939–952 (1990).

42. Neuenschwander, S., Castelo-Branco, M., Baron, J., and Singer, W. Feed-forward synchronization: propagation of temporal patterns along the retinothalamocortical pathway. *Philos. Trans. R. Soc. Lond. B Biol. Sci.* 357, 1869–1876 (2002).

43. Whittington, M. A., Traub, R. D., and Jefferys, J. G. Synchronized oscillations in interneuron networks driven by metabotropic glutamate receptor activation. *Nature* 373, 612–615 (1995).

44. Penttonen, M., Kamondi, A., Acsady, L., and Buzsaki, G. Gamma frequency oscillation in the hippocampus of the rat: intracellular analysis in vivo. *Eur. J. Neurosci.* 10, 718–728 (1998).

45. Whittington, M. A., Traub, R. D., Kopell, N., Ermentrout, B., and Buhl, E. H. Inhibition-based rhythms: experimental and mathematical observations on network dynamics. *Int. J. Psychophysiol.* 38, 315–336 (2000).

46. Bacci, A., Rudolph, U., Huguenard, J. R., and Prince, D. A. Major differences in inhibitory synaptic transmission onto two neocortical interneuron subclasses. *J. Neurosci.* 23, 9664–9674 (2003).

47. Shadlen, M. N., and Movshon, J. A. Synchrony unbound: a critical evaluation of the temporal binding hypothesis. *Neuron* 24, 67–77, 111–125 (1999). (This review argues that synchrony does not play an important role in binding the responses of neurons. The article states that synchrony cannot be used as an informational code.)

48. Azouz, R., and Gray, C. M. Adaptive coincidence detection and dynamic gain control in visual cortical neurons in vivo. *Neuron* 37, 513–523 (2003). (References 48 and 49 show how true synchrony, due to neurons responding to the same object, can be distinguished from background synchrony due to high firing rates. They show that the spiking threshold is an adaptive function of firing rate.)

49. Azouz, R., and Gray, C. M. Dynamic spike threshold reveals a mechanism for synaptic coincidence detection in cortical neurons in vivo. *Proc. Natl. Acad. Sci. USA* 97, 8110–8115 (2000). (References 48 and 49 show how true synchrony, due to neurons responding to the same object, can be distinguished from background synchrony due to high firing rates. They show that the spiking threshold is an adaptive function of firing rate.)

50. Wang, Z., Xu, N. L., Wu, C. P., Duan, S., and Poo, M. M. Bidirectional changes in spatial dendritic integration accompanying long-term synaptic modifications. *Neuron* 37, 463–472 (2003).

51. Shadlen, M. N., and Newsome, W. T. The variable discharge of cortical neurons: implications for connectivity, computation, and information coding. *J. Neurosci.* 18, 3870–3896 (1998). (References 51 and 52 argue that neurons are intrinsically noisy and therefore cannot reliably transmit a temporal code.)

52. Shadlen, M. N., and Newsome, W. T. Noise, neural codes and cortical organization. *Curr. Opin. Neurobiol.* 4, 569–579 (1994). (References 51 and 52 argue that neurons are intrinsically noisy and therefore cannot reliably transmit a temporal code.)

53. Mazurek, M. E., and Shadlen, M. N. Limits to the temporal fidelity of cortical spike rate signals. *Nat. Neurosci.* 5, 463–471 (2002).

54. Abbott, L. F., and Dayan, P. The effect of correlated variability on the accuracy of a population code. *Neural Comput.* 11, 91–101 (1999).

55. Kenyon, G. T., Theiler, J., George, J. S., Travis, B. J., and Marshak, D. W. Correlated firing improves stimulus discrimination in a retinal model. *Neural Comput.* 16, 2261–2291 (2004).

56. Kenyon, G. T., et al. A model of high-frequency oscillatory potentials in retinal ganglion cells. *Vis. Neurosci.* 20, 465–480 (2003). (Presents a synchronously oscillatory model of the retina that is used in Reference 57.)

57. Kenyon, G. T., and Marshak, D. W. Gap junctions with amacrine cells provide a feedback pathway for ganglion cells within the retina. *Proc. R. Soc. Lond. B Biol. Sci.* 265, 919–925 (1998). (Uses the model from Reference 56 to investigate the role that different neurons in the retina play in retinal oscillations.)

58. Samonds, J. M., and Bonds, A. B. Gamma oscillation maintains stimulus structure-dependent synchronization in cat visual cortex. *J. Neurophysiol.* 93, 223–236 (2005).

59. Laurent, G., Wehr, M., and Davidowitz, H. Temporal representations of odors in an olfactory network. *J. Neurosci.* 16, 3837–3847 (1996).

60. Friedrich, R. W., and Stopfer, M. Recent dynamics in olfactory population coding. *Curr. Opin. Neurobiol.* 11, 468–474 (2001).

61. Laurent, G. Olfactory network dynamics and the coding of multidimensional signals. *Nat. Rev. Neurosci.* 3, 884–895 (2002). (An excellent review of the role of temporal coding in the olfactory system.)

62. Huerta, R., Nowotny, T., Garcia-Sanchez, M., Abarbanel, H. D., and Rabinovich, M. I. Learning classification in the olfactory system of insects. *Neural. Comput.* 16, 1601–1640 (2004).

63. Zola-Morgan, S., and Squire, L. R. Medial temporal lesions in monkeys impair memory on a variety of tasks sensitive to human amnesia. *Behav. Neurosci.* 99, 22–34 (1985).

64. Zola-Morgan, S., and Squire, L. R. Memory impairment in monkeys following lesions limited to the hippocampus. *Behav. Neurosci.* 100, 155–160 (1986).

65. Eichenbaum, H. A cortical-hippocampal system for declarative memory. *Nat. Rev. Neurosci.* 1, 41–50 (2000).

66. McNaughton, B. L., Barnes, C. A., and O'Keefe, J. The contributions of position, direction, and velocity to single unit activity in the hippocampus of freely-moving rats. *Exp. Brain Res.* 52, 41–49 (1983).

67. Ferbinteanu, J., and Shapiro, M. L. Prospective and retrospective memory coding in the hippocampus. *Neuron* 40, 1227–1239 (2003).

68. Bland, B. H., and Oddie, S. D. Theta band oscillation and synchrony in the hippocampal formation and associated structures: the case for its role in sensorimotor integration. *Behav. Brain Res.* 127, 119–136 (2001).

69. Jensen, O., and Lisman, J. E. Novel lists of 7 ± 2 known items can be reliably stored in an oscillatory short-term memory network: interaction with long-term memory. *Learn. Mem.* 3, 257–263 (1996).

70. Jensen, O., and Lisman, J. E. Theta/gamma networks with slow NMDA channels learn sequences and encode episodic memory: role of NMDA channels in recall. *Learn. Mem.* 3, 264–278 (1996).

71. Jensen, O., and Lisman, J. E. An oscillatory short-term memory buffer model can account for data on the Sternberg task. *J. Neurosci.* 18, 10688–10699 (1998).

72. Lisman, J. E., and Otmakhova, N. A. Storage, recall, and novelty detection of sequences by the hippocampus: elaborating on the SOCRATIC model to account for normal and aberrant effects of dopamine. *Hippocampus* 11, 551–568 (2001).

73. Lisman, J. E., and Idiart, M. A. Storage of 7 ± 2 short-term memories in oscillatory subcycles. *Science* 267, 1512–1515 (1995). (Presents a model of how theta and gamma oscillations can encode short-term memories.)

74. Miller, G. The magical number seven plus or minus two: Some limits on our capacity for processing information. *Psychol. Rev.* 63, 81–97 (1956).

75. Lawrie, S. M., et al. Reduced frontotemporal functional connectivity in schizophrenia associated with auditory hallucinations. *Biol. Psychiatry* 51, 1008–1011 (2002).

76. Just, M. A., Cherkassky, V. L., Keller, T. A., and Minshew, N. J. Cortical activation and synchronization during sentence comprehension in high-functioning autism: evidence of underconnectivity. *Brain* 127, 1811–1821 (2004).

77. Hubel, D. H., and Wiesel, T. N. Receptive fields of optic nerve fibres in the spider monkey. *J. Physiol.* 154, 572–580 (1960). (References 77 and 78 present the pioneering work of Hubel and Wiesel in investigating the responses of V1 cortical cells to stimuli. They established what is now the classical receptive field of these neurons.)

78. Hubel, D. H., and Wiesel, T. N. Receptive fields of single neurones in the cat's striate cortex. *J. Physiol.* 148, 574–591 (1959). (References 77 and 78 present the pioneering work of Hubel and Wiesel in investigating the responses of V1 cortical cells to stimuli. They established what is now the classical receptive field of these neurons.)

79. Yen, S. C., and Finkel, L. H. Extraction of perceptually salient contours by striate cortical networks. *Vision Res.* 38, 719–741 (1998).

80. Engel, A. K., and Singer, W. Temporal binding and the neural correlates of sensory awareness. *Trends Cogn. Sci.* 5, 16–25 (2001).

81. Schneider, G. Neural networks are useful tools for drug design. *Neural Networks* 13, 15–16 (2000).

82. Schneider, G., and Wrede, P. Artificial neural networks for computer-based molecular design. *Prog. Biophys. Mol. Biol.* 70, 175–222 (1998).

83. Hopfield, J. J., Brody, C. D., and Roweis, S. In *Advances in Neural Information Processing Systems* (Jordan, M., Kearns, M., and Solla, S., Eds.), MIT Press, Denver, CO, 1998, 166–172.

84. Hopfield, J. J. Pattern recognition computation using action potential timing for stimulus representation. *Nature* 376, 33–36 (1995).

85. Abarbanel, H. D., Huerta, R., and Rabinovich, M. I. Dynamical model of long-term synaptic plasticity. *Proc. Natl. Acad. Sci. USA* 99, 10132–10137 (2002).

86. Nowotny, T., Zhigulin, V. P., Selverston, A. I., Abarbanel, H. D., and Rabinovich, M. I. Enhancement of synchronization in a hybrid neural circuit by spike-timing dependent plasticity. *J. Neurosci.* 23, 9776–9785 (2003).

87. Markram, H., and Tsodyks, M. Redistribution of synaptic efficacy between neocortical pyramidal neurons. *Nature* 382, 807–810 (1996).

88. Forsythe, I. D., and Westbrook, G. L. Slow excitatory postsynaptic currents mediated by N-methyl-D-aspartate receptors on cultured mouse central neurones. *J. Physiol.* 396, 515–533 (1988).

89. Mainen, Z. F., and Sejnowski, T. J. Reliability of spike timing in neocortical neurons. *Science* 268, 1503–1506 (1995).

90. Alonso, J. M., Usrey, W. M., and Reid, R. C. Precisely correlated firing in cells of the lateral geniculate nucleus. *Nature* 383, 815–819 (1996).

91. Bi, G., and Poo, M. Synaptic modification by correlated activity: Hebb's postulate revisited. *Annu. Rev. Neurosci.* 24, 139–166 (2001).

92. Buracas, G. T., Zador, A. M., DeWeese, M. R., and Albright, T. D. Efficient discrimination of temporal patterns by motion-sensitive neurons in primate visual cortex. *Neuron* 20, 959–969 (1998).

93. Kapetanovic, I. M., Rosenfeld, S., and Izmirlian, G. Overview of commonly used bioinformatics methods and their applications. *Ann. NY Acad. Sci.* 1020, 10–21 (2004).

94. Dayhoff, J. E., and DeLeo, J. M. Artificial neural networks: opening the black box. *Cancer* 91, 1615–1635 (2001).

95. Qian, N., and Sejnowski, T. J. Predicting the secondary structure of globular proteins using neural network models. *J. Mol. Biol.* 202, 865–884 (1988).

96. Adamczak, R., Porollo, A., and Meller, J. Accurate prediction of solvent accessibility using neural networks-based regression. *Proteins* 56, 753–767 (2004).

97. Barnden, J. A., and Chady, M. In *Handbook of Brain Theory and Neural Networks* (Arbib, M. A., Ed.), MIT Press, Cambridge, MA, 2003, 113–117. (The book has a wealth of information regarding computational approaches to understanding neural computation.)

98. Arbib, M. A. In *Handbook of Brain Theory and Neural Networks* (Arbib, M. A., Ed.), MIT Press, Cambridge, MA, 2003, 44–47. (The book has a wealth of information regarding computational approaches to understanding neural computation.)

99. Stephens, G. J., Neuenschwander, S., George, J. S., Singer, W., and Kenyon, G. T. See globally, spike locally: oscillations in a retinal model encode large visual features. *Biol. Cybern.* 95, 327–348 (2006).

3 Using Pharmacodynamic Biomarkers to Accelerate Early Clinical Drug Development

Ole Vesterqvist

CONTENTS

INTRODUCTION

Pharmaceutical companies are increasingly using biomarkers (biological markers) in early clinical drug development (phase I) to enable early proof-of-concept studies and to better predict the dose range for phases II and III. The average success rate from first-in-human (also called "first-in-man") to registration was about 11% for all therapeutic areas during a ten-year period for ten of the big pharmaceutical companies.[1] A major cause of attrition in the clinical phases in 2000 was a lack of efficacy, and there is obviously a need to provide better and more meaningful data to assess the efficacy of compounds in early clinical development.

Biomarkers play an important role in decision making during the early phases of clinical drug development. Many biomarkers are used to assess the safety of a drug; others are used to study the pharmacologic effects related to the mechanism of action. The pharmacodynamic (PD) biomarker data can be used with the pharmacokinetic

(PK) data to show a relationship between the drug concentrations and the drug effects or side effects as measured by the PD biomarker. The PK/PD relationship can then support decision making regarding dose and dose regimen.

Very few biomarkers, e.g., HIV plasma viral load, blood pressure, and cholesterol, have reached the level of surrogate end points substituting for clinical end points.[2] There is currently no regulatory guidance for method development and validation of the "research"-type of biomarkers, i.e., the nondiagnostic biomarkers. Nor is there any guidance for the appropriate use of research biomarkers in drug development. Most of the PD biomarkers used in early clinical drug development belong to this class, and many challenges are associated with using PD biomarkers in early clinical drug development. Validation (performance assessment) of the biomarker methods is only part of the challenge; choosing the right biomarker or set of biomarkers is another. Biomarker results in early clinical drug development are mostly used for internal business decision making, with limited regulatory guidance. The level of validation of the PD biomarkers and their associated methods is basically up to each user to define. The intended use of a biomarker or a set of biomarkers in early clinical drug development will, therefore, to a great extent, dictate the validation of the biomarkers and associated methods.[3] To successfully use PD biomarkers in early clinical drug development, it is imperative to have cross-functional biomarker teams define the purpose for each individual biomarker or set of biomarkers.

PHARMACODYNAMIC BIOMARKERS

A PD biomarker has been defined as a characteristic that is objectively measured and evaluated as an indicator of pharmacologic responses to a therapeutic intervention.[2] Biological markers have been used for centuries in evaluating PD effects of drugs. Aspirin (acetylsalicylic acid), synthesized in 1897 by Felix Hoffman at the Bayer company in Germany, is undoubtedly the most used drug in the world.[4] The history of aspirin is a lesson in the use of PD biomarkers to study the PD effects of a drug.

Fever was one of the first PD biomarkers used to evaluate the effects of salicylates, and in about 1757, after six years of clinical observations, the Rev. Mr. Edmund Stone proposed that willow bark be used in febrile disorders.[5] Fever was also a biomarker in the early studies of the effects of aspirin on humans in the 19th century. However, the mechanism of action of aspirin would remain unknown until 1971, when three reports in the same issue of the journal *Nature New Biology* demonstrated that the inhibition of prostaglandins was the mechanism of action of aspirin and aspirinlike compounds.[6–8] In these papers, the biomarker was "prostaglandin-like activity" measured by a bioassay using isolated stomach strips and colons from rat. The discovery of prostaglandins and the use of bioassays to determine the presence of prostaglandins in tissue supernatants were essential in providing the tools to reveal the mechanism of action of aspirin.

The development of new analytical technologies and the isolation of the active enzyme, cyclooxygenase, in 1976, gave scientists new insights into the PD effects of aspirin.[9] The long-lasting (up to 10 days) PD effects of aspirin on platelets was revealed from studies of the acetylation of cyclooxygenase on human platelets.[10] Aspirin irreversibly inhibits cyclooxygenase, and for the nonnucleated platelets, this can mean lifelong inhibition of cyclooxygenase. With the discovery of thromboxane A_2 and the introduction of isotope-dilution quantitative gas chromatography–mass spectrometry methods for measurement of urinary metabolites of thromboxane B_2 in the 1980s, the long-lasting (up to 10 days) PD effect on platelets was confirmed in clinical studies.[11,12] These findings explained why a 325-mg aspirin dose given every other day caused a prolonged inhibition of platelet thromboxane formation and a 44% reduction in the risk of myocardial infarction in healthy physicians.[13] Interestingly, this intermittent dose of aspirin did not cause any significant increased risk in gastrointestinal discomfort, a major side effect of aspirin, suggesting that the gastrointestinal PD effects of aspirin are relatively short lasting compared with the cardiovascular effects.[13]

The PD effect of a high dose (1 g) of aspirin on the biosynthesis of prostacyclin (measured as urinary excretion of 2,3-dinor-6-keto-prostaglandin $F_{1\alpha}$, the major urinary metabolite of prostacyclin), a potent vasodilator and inhibitor of platelet aggregation, in endothelial cells was of much shorter duration (3–4 h) than the PD effect on platelet thromboxane A_2 biosynthesis (Figure 3.1).[14] These findings suggested that endothelial cells, which are nucleated, are capable of synthesizing new and active cyclooxygenase as soon as aspirin is metabolized. The short-lasting

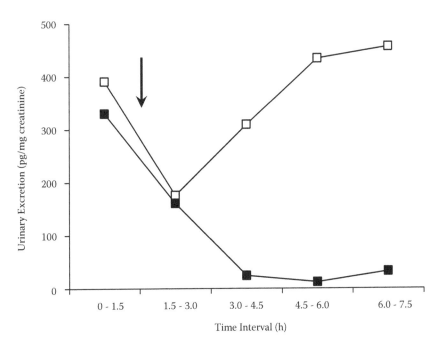

FIGURE 3.1 Effects of 1 g of aspirin on the urinary excretion of 2,3-dinor-TxB$_2$ (closed symbols) and 2,3-dinor-6-keto-PGF$_{1\alpha}$ (open symbols), the major urinary metabolites of thromboxane A$_2$ and prostacyclin, in a healthy volunteer. *Arrow* indicates aspirin administration time. (From Vesterqvist, O. *Eur. J. Clin. Pharmacol.* 1986, 30: 69–73. With permission.)

inhibition of prostacyclin was difficult to interpret until the cyclooxygenase-2 (COX-2) isoform was discovered in 1991.[15] Later clinical studies of celecoxib, a specific COX-2 inhibitor, showed a selective inhibition of the urinary excretion of the prostacyclin metabolite, 2,3-dinor-6-keto-prostaglandin $F_{1\alpha}$, in healthy volunteers for up to 24 hours after dosing.[16] This suggested that COX-2 is a major source of systemic prostacyclin biosynthesis in healthy humans and, considering that the half-life of aspirin is only about 17 minutes compared with a half-life of celecoxib of about 11 hours, one might speculate that the short-lasting inhibition of prostacyclin biosynthesis by high doses of aspirin is due to its inhibition of COX-2.[17]

The discovery of a third isoform of cyclooxygenase in 2002, COX-3, has further increased our understanding of the mechanism of action of aspirin and other fever-reducing drugs.[18] The discovery of the COX-3 isoform also explained the observation made 13 years earlier that acetaminophen causes a pronounced inhibition of prostacyclin biosynthesis in humans.[19]

The history of aspirin teaches us that the field of PD biomarkers is full of adjustments. Our knowledge of biology and biochemistry is constantly changing and challenges our previous interpretations of biomarker results. With improved analytical technologies and methods, PD biomarker measurements can be performed more accurately and precisely, allowing for statistically significant detection of PD changes that are smaller in magnitude and that are observed in clinical studies with fewer subjects. Improvements in assay performance often lead to a reevaluation of the value of specific biomarkers. C-reactive protein (CRP) is an example of this. The development of the high-sensitivity method for C-reactive protein made it possible to measure CRP at much lower concentrations with improved reproducibility, and this allowed clinical investigators to reevaluate CRP as a predictive marker for cardiovascular risk.[20]

PHARMACODYNAMIC BIOMARKER METHOD VALIDATION

The majority of published papers outlining method validation (performance assessment) parameters (e.g., precision, accuracy, and concentration–response relationship) have focused on method validation in analytical laboratories that support measurements of drugs.[21,22] Most analytical laboratories involved with the development and measurement of PD biomarkers are familiar with these validation parameters, and many laboratories document the validation of biomarker methods in a formal report.[3,23,24] The nondiagnostic PD biomarker assays are currently not regulated, and the U.S. Food and Drug Administration (FDA) has not issued any detailed guidelines and criteria for performance assessment of the PD biomarker methods. The current FDA Guidance for Industry (Exposure–Response Relationship: Study Design, Data Analysis, and Regulatory Applications) states that "many biomarkers will never undergo the rigorous statistical evaluations that would establish their value as a surrogate end point to determine efficacy and safety, but they can still have use in drug development and regulatory decision making."[25] It is therefore up to the analytical laboratories to set their own recommendations and standards for the performance assessment of the PD biomarker methods. Some of the recommended validation parameters for assessing the performance of PD biomarker methods are listed in Table 3.1.

TABLE 3.1
Recommended Parameters for Validation of PD Biomarker Methods

Validation Parameters	Description
Quality of biomarker calibrators/standards	Evaluate the quality of reference material
Calibration/standard curve	Evaluate relationship between known quantities (concentration, enzyme activity, number of cells, etc.) of biomarker reference material in artificial/true matrix and measured instrument response
Accuracy	Evaluate the closeness of the measured value and the "true" value
Analytical specificity	Evaluate the ability of the method to measure the biomarker without reacting with other related substances
Imprecision	Evaluate the variability in replicate measurements (intra- and interassay)
Analytical range	Establish analytical range of the biomarker over which the method shows acceptable performance
Reportable range	Establish range of reportable results over which the method is validated (may exceed analytical range when samples are diluted or concentrated)
Sample stability	Evaluate stability of biomarker in the sample matrix under conditions that mimic the study conditions
Ruggedness	Evaluate the method performance when using different analysts and different batches of reagents over a longer period of time

The FDA Guidance for Method Validation (Bioanalytical Methods Used for Nonhuman Pharmacology/Toxicology Studies and Preclinical Studies) has taken the approach that "one size fits all" by setting fixed criteria for acceptance of method performance.[26] However, this approach will not work for biomarker methods in general. The ICH Harmonized Tripartite Guideline states that "the main objective of validation of an analytical procedure is to demonstrate that the procedure is suitable for its intended use."[27] This is especially true for PD biomarkers, where each biomarker method, depending on the intended use, can require its own performance acceptance criteria. The proficiency testing criteria for acceptable performance of diagnostic tests are specific to each test and are quite variable; for example, the acceptable performance for chloride and albumin is ±5% and ±10%, respectively, but is ±30% for creatine kinase and amylase.[28] Validation for biomarker methods tends to be more complicated than that for drug assays, and it is often not possible to evaluate all of the validation parameters outlined in the FDA Guidance for Method Validation.[26] Contributing to the complexity and difficulty of establishing standards is the fact that biomarkers are measured using a diversity of technology platforms, such as liquid chromatography–mass spectrometry, immunoassays, flow cytometry, quantitative reverse-transcription polymerase chain reaction, immunohistochemistry, etc.

One of the main objectives of the method-performance evaluation process is to characterize (Table 3.1) and control sources of variability. Too much emphasis is often given to prespecified method-performance criteria. For example, a PD biomarker method showing an imprecision of 30–40% CV (coefficient of variation) at low concentrations of the biomarker measured in specimens collected prior to dosing can be acceptable if (a) the PD effects of the drug lead to a tenfold increase in the concentrations and (b) the imprecision of the assay at these concentrations is below 10% CV. Determination of the absolute accuracy of a biomarker assay can be very challenging. This is especially true for many proteins where well-characterized reference materials/standards or reference methods may not be available.

A major challenge in evaluating the performance of a PD biomarker method is the fact that, until the first-in-human study is conducted, we do not know what the actual PD effects will be on the biomarker in humans. It is therefore difficult to predict how sensitive and precise the biomarker method needs to be to enable detection of any PD effects. PD biomarker results from preclinical *in vivo* drug studies can, to some extent, be used to predict the effects of the drug on the PD biomarker, and this is further discussed later in this chapter (see section entitled "Early Clinical Drug Development").

Once the method performance has been characterized, a comprehensive method validation report should be issued. To control for changes in method performance, laboratories use quality control (QC) samples. The QC samples should, whenever possible, be based on the true matrix and acceptance criteria (usually mean ±2 SD or the 95% confidence interval) determined based on the actual interassay variability in the laboratory performing the assay during the clinical study. The QC samples should also cover the range of expected values (concentrations, activity, cell number, etc.).

The FDA Guidance for Method Validation recommends that the number of QC samples be in multiples of three, at three different concentrations, and that "at least 67% (4 out of 6) of QC samples should be within 15% of their respective nominal value."[26] It is interesting that this recommendation does not take into account that many assays can perform with an interassay imprecision far better than ±15%. For example, if an assay shows an interassay (interday) imprecision of ±4% CV, the QC sample of a particular run could be outside the mean ±3.5 SD and still be acceptable with a rule of within ±15% of nominal value. However, the use of a predefined value of, for example, ±15% of nominal value for accepting QC sample results is not recommended for PD biomarkers. For frequently used PD biomarker methods, the use of the Westgard "multirule" procedure is recommended.[28] This procedure uses a series of control rules based on mean ±2 SD, ±3 SD, and ±4 SD, for interpreting the QC results as well as for keeping the probability for false rejections low. For less frequently used methods, it is recommended that (a) the acceptance criteria be based on a mean ±2 SD range or the 95% confidence interval of the actual interassay variability and (b) at least 67% (two out of three) of the QC samples (minimum three samples of three divergently different concentrations, activities, etc., per analytical run) should be within this range of their respective nominal values to accept an analytical run.

A more accurate picture of the actual performance of the assay during the study can be determined by depicting the performance of the quality controls during a clinical study, and this picture can differ somewhat from the performance characteristics obtained during method validation. The information regarding actual assay performance (sometimes called in-study validation) will undoubtedly improve interpretation of the biomarker results generated in early clinical drug development. QC samples can also play an important role whenever multiple laboratories are used to provide the analytical service. The use of multiple laboratories is common whenever multiple clinical sites are involved in a clinical study or when the biomarkers require analysis within hours of sampling due to instability or other preanalytical restrictions pertinent to the particular biomarkers. In this case, the postanalysis QC results from one laboratory (the "reference laboratory") can be used as reference values against which the results from the other laboratories will be normalized or adjusted. This allows for statistical analysis of all results combined when the QC results have been shown to meet certain standards.

PHARMACODYNAMIC BIOMARKER EVALUATION

To use PD biomarkers optimally in early clinical development, we need to define their roles and build a consensus on the utility of the PD biomarkers in decision making. We need to evaluate (validate) not only the analytical methods, but also the biomarkers. Low-density lipoprotein (LDL) cholesterol and HIV viral load are examples of clinical biomarkers that can guide therapeutic development. It takes a long time and a lot of effort to evaluate clinical biomarkers for diagnostic or therapeutic purposes, and as long as we are using these biomarkers in clinical studies, they will continuously undergo evaluation. This ongoing evaluation will often change our understanding of how a particular biomarker can play a role in making diagnostic and therapeutic decisions.

The diagnostic biomarkers are unquestionably the most extensively evaluated biomarkers. They undergo continuous evaluation with regard to their sensitivity (number of subjects with disease correctly identified using the biomarker among all subjects with disease, i.e., detection of disease when disease is truly present) and specificity (number of subjects without disease correctly identified using the biomarker among all subjects without disease, i.e., recognition of disease absence when the disease is truly absent). However, they are not always "perfect" biomarkers. For example, prostate-specific antigen (PSA), measured as free, total, or complexed PSA, is a commonly used tumor biomarker in oncology, but it shows relatively poor specificity (14–51%) despite a 92% sensitivity.[29]

Evaluation of a PD biomarker is a process that starts in drug discovery, when potential drug candidates have been identified, and continues when the PD biomarker is used in clinical studies. During this evaluation process, it is key to characterize the biological variability and to identify other potential preanalytical sources of variability in the measured biomarker (Table 3.2). The variability in biomarker measurements caused by biological/preanalytical factors is usually greater than the variability caused by analytical factors.

In drug discovery, measurements of biomarkers should preferably be performed *in vivo* in animal models, but *in vitro/ex vivo* studies using, for example, human whole blood or blood cells can also be useful. The more closely the sampling procedure in the preclinical model mimics the clinical situation, the better is the result. The PD biomarker evaluation process in drug discovery should, in detail, characterize the PD effects on the biomarker and correlate these to the PK results. Once the drug is transferred into clinical drug development, further evaluation of

TABLE 3.2
Sources of Biological and Preanalytical Variability
in Biomarker Measurements

Sources	Examples
Specimen collection	Site of collection
	Plasma versus serum
	Time of venous occlusion
	Type of anticoagulant
	Type of preservative
Specimen handling and storage	Maintenance of specimen identification
	Transportation temperature
	Time of transportation
	Storage temperature
	Time of storage
Age, gender, and race	Males and females
	Whites, Blacks, Native Americans
Posture	Ambulatory, upright, supine
Exercise	Duration and intensity of the activity
Food intake/diet	Time of food intake relative to specimen collection
	Vegetarianism, fasting, malnutrition
Circadian variation	Cyclical variations during the day
Seasonal and long-term cyclical variation	Seasonal dietary and physical activity changes
	Menstrual cycle

the sources of biological variation in humans should take place prior to the first-in-human studies. The clinical biomarker evaluation provides valuable information about the total variation (biological plus analytical) in the biomarker.

EARLY CLINICAL DRUG DEVELOPMENT

A key objective in early clinical drug development is to establish the relationship between dose and the PD effects. The use of PD biomarkers can accelerate early clinical drug development by providing valuable information verifying the mechanism of action and demonstrating dose- and time-dependent PD effects. This information will support dose selection for phase II. If there is no effect on the PD biomarkers at any of the doses tested in phase I, the biomarker results can support a no-go decision to end clinical development.

Biomarkers can objectively be measured to study the PD effects of drugs; for example, the enzymatic activity of angiotensin-converting enzyme (ACE) and the concentration of angiotensin I and II can be measured in plasma to study PD effects of ACE inhibitors.[30] The PD biomarkers play an important role in the first clinical studies of a new drug. In these studies, under controlled conditions, the PD biomarkers allow us to study the dynamic effects of a drug. In most first-in-human studies, healthy subjects are used to evaluate drug safety. In these studies, the PD

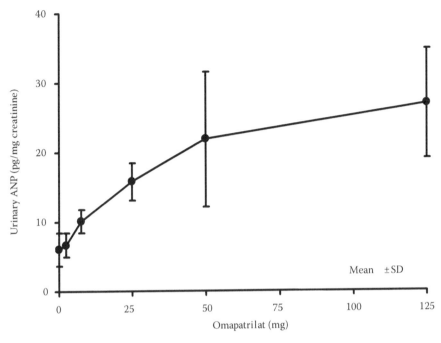

FIGURE 3.2 Effects of ascending single doses of omapatrilat on the urinary excretion of atrial natriuretic peptide (ANP) in healthy subjects. (From Vesterqvist, O., and Reeves, R.A. *Curr. Hypertens. Rep.* 2001; 3[Suppl. 2]: 22–27. With permission.)

biomarker results provide valuable information about the duration and magnitude of the PD effects (Figure 3.2),[31] especially as the clinical end points may not be meaningful to study in a healthy population. Together with the PK data, the PD biomarker results will be important in establishing the dose and dose regimen for further clinical studies in a patient population.

TRANSITIONING OF PHARMACODYNAMIC BIOMARKERS FROM DISCOVERY TO DEVELOPMENT

Most potential PD biomarkers are identified in the discovery phase of drug development. One of the biggest challenges in choosing the right PD biomarkers is the successful translation of these biomarkers from preclinical to clinical development. The initial validation of the value of a PD biomarker will therefore come from preclinical studies using *in vivo* animal models or from *ex vivo* studies using either animal or human samples. However, animal models often do not predict human biology, and many of the PD biomarker methods that are used in preclinical laboratories have gone through only limited analytical validation and characterization. It is, therefore, important that potential PD biomarkers be identified early in the research and development process to allow adequate time to validate the biomarker methods and also to define the intended use of the biomarkers prior to the start of

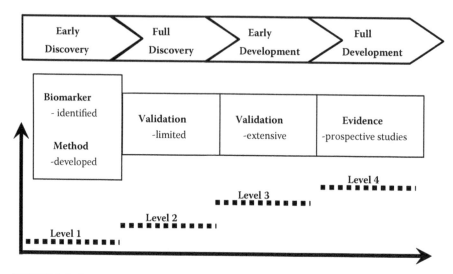

FIGURE 3.3 Staged approach to biomarker validation in drug discovery and development.

the phase I clinical studies. PD biomarker results from preclinical *in vivo* drug studies can be used to predict the PD effects of the drug on the biomarkers in the early clinical studies.

As a biomarker is used in early and full (late) drug discovery and eventually in clinical drug development, the level of biomarker validation can be addressed with a staged approach (Figure 3.3). For each level, the extent of validation and the confidence level in the PD biomarker are concomitantly increased. The intended use of a PD biomarker or a set of PD biomarkers in early clinical drug development will, to a great extent, dictate the evaluation of the biomarkers and the validation of the associated methods. However, there is limited time to develop and validate clinical biomarker methods and to evaluate the potential PD biomarkers prior to the initiation of phase I studies. The time available for method validation will limit the extent of the validation/evaluation, and this limitation has to be acknowledged by the clinical drug development teams.

USING PHARMACODYNAMIC BIOMARKERS IN EARLY CLINICAL DRUG DEVELOPMENT

The analytical validation of biomarker methods is often performed in an environment that differs from the one in which the methods will be performed during the clinical studies. In addition, analysts other than those who performed the method validation may perform the analysis of specimens from the clinical studies. Therefore, method performance during the actual analysis of clinical specimens may differ from that observed during assay validation.

Many of the preanalytical variables that challenge data interpretation can be addressed in the study design. Clinical studies can be designed to minimize the effects of preanalytical sources of variability, such as effects of posture, exercise, diurnal

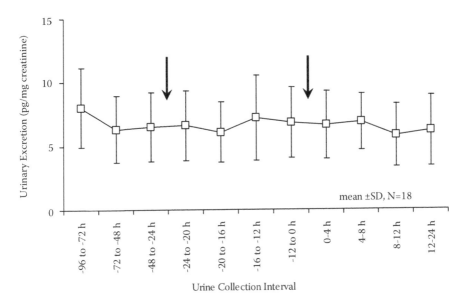

FIGURE 3.4 Urinary excretion of atrial natriuretic peptide (ANP) in placebo-treated healthy subjects in a phase I study. At a mean individual urinary excretion of ANP ranging from 3.1 to 13.8 pg/mg creatinine, the overall intrasubject variability in the urinary excretion was 22% ± 9% CV (mean ± SD, $N = 18$) and a range from 10% to 45% CV. *Arrows* indicate placebo administration time. (From unpublished data provided by Bristol–Myers Squibb Company. With permission.)

biorhythms, and food intake. The use of a placebo group will give valuable information on the total variability in the PD biomarker results: the sum of the biological and analytical errors (Figure 3.4).

To support decision making in early clinical drug development, it is absolutely necessary that the PD biomarker results be delivered in a timely fashion. New multiplexing technologies and improved automation have enabled laboratories to quickly provide measurements of many PD biomarkers in a single study. The management of the enormous quantities of data alone can become a rate-limiting factor, and there is a need for efficient bioinformatics solutions. These solutions must include data storage, management, and analysis as well as a predefined process for providing the PD biomarker results to the clinical team. This is especially important in the single and multiple ascending dose studies, where timely information about the PD biomarker results following each dose group can give the clinical team additional and valuable time to prepare and plan for upcoming phase II and III clinical studies.

CONCLUSION

Despite advances in basic science and recent breakthroughs in biomedical research, the industry has not been able to improve the identification of successful drug candidates. The average success rate from first-in-human studies to registration is about 11%.[1] The FDA has recognized the most pressing drug development problems and has created a list of critical-path opportunities.[32] Part of the goals of the critical-path research includes the development of new scientific and technical tools, including biomarkers and assays, that will make the development process more efficient and effective.[32] Pharmacodynamic biomarkers have long been used and will continue to be used in early clinical drug development. The road ahead will likely lead to the incorporation of more PD biomarkers in drug discovery using analytically validated methods. The ultimate goal for the use of PD biomarkers in early clinical drug development is to enable rapid evaluation of new drug candidates in humans and to support decision making. This can be accomplished only if the objectives and expectations for using the PD biomarkers are clearly defined up front.

REFERENCES

1. Kola, I., and Landis, J. Can the pharmaceutical industry reduce attrition rates? *Nat. Rev. Drug Discov.* 2004; 3: 711–715.
2. Biomarker Definitions Working Group. Biomarkers and surrogate endpoints: preferred definitions and conceptual framework. *Clin. Pharmacol. Ther.* 2001; 69: 89–95.
3. Swanson, B. Delivery of high-quality biomarker assays. *Disease Markers* 2002; 18: 47–56.
4. Vane, J.R. The mechanism of action of aspirin. *Thromb. Res.* 2003; 110: 255–258.
5. Weissman, G. Aspirin. *Sci. Am.* 1991; January: 84–90.
6. Vane, J.R. Inhibition of prostaglandin synthesis is a mechanism of action for aspirin-like drugs. *Nature (New Biol.)* 1971; 231: 232–235.
7. Smith, J.B., and Willis, A.L. Aspirin selectively inhibits prostaglandin production in human platelets. *Nature (New Biol.)* 1971; 231: 235–237.
8. Ferreira, S.H., Moncada, S., and Vane, J.R. Indomethacin and aspirin abolish prostaglandin release from the spleen. *Nature (New Biol.)* 1971; 231: 237–239.
9. Hemler, M., Lands, W.E.M., and Smith, W.L. Purification of the cyclooxygenase that forms prostaglandins: demonstration of two forms of iron in the holoenzyme. *J. Biol. Chem.* 1976; 251: 5575–5579.
10. Burch, J.W., Stanford, N., and Majerus, P.W. Inhibition of platelet prostaglandin synthetase by oral aspirin. *J. Clin. Invest.* 1978; 61: 314–319.
11. Hamberg, M., Svensson, J., and Samuelsson, B. Thromboxanes: a new group of biologically active compounds derived from prostaglandin endoperoxides. *Proc. Natl. Acad. Sci. USA* 1975; 72: 2994–2998.
12. Vesterqvist, O., and Gréen, K. Urinary excretion of 2,3-dinor-thromboxane B_2 in man under normal conditions, following drugs and during some pathological conditions. *Prostaglandins* 1984, 27: 627–644.
13. Steering Committee of Physicians' Health Study Research Group. Final report on the aspirin component of the ongoing physicians' health study. *N. Engl. J. Med.* 1989; 321: 129–135.
14. Vesterqvist, O. Rapid recovery of in vivo prostacyclin formation after inhibition by aspirin: evidence from measurements of the major urinary metabolite of prostacyclin by GC-MS. *Eur. J. Clin. Pharmacol.* 1986, 30: 69–73.
15. Xie, W.L., Chipman, J.G., Robertson, D.L., Eriksson, R.L., and Simmons, D.L. Expression of a mitogen-responsive gene encoding prostaglandin synthase is regulated by mRNA splicing. *Proc. Natl. Acad. Sci. USA* 1991; 88: 2692–2696.

16. McAdam, B.F., Catella-Lawson, F., Mardini, I.A., Kapoor, S., Lawson, J.A., and FitzGerald, G.A. Systemic biosynthesis of prostacyclin by cyclooxygenase (COX)-2: the human pharmacology of a selective inhibitor of COX-2. *Proc. Natl. Acad. Sci. USA* 1999; 96: 272–277.

17. Davies, N.M., McLachlan, A.J., Day, R.O., and Williams, K.M. Clinical pharmacokinetics and pharmacodynamics of Celecoxib. *Clin. Pharmacokinet.* 2000; 38: 225–242.

18. Chandrasekharan, N.V., Dai, H., Roos, K.L., Evanson, N.K., Tomsik, J., Elton, T.S., and Simmons, D.L. *Proc. Natl. Acad. Sci. USA* 2002; 99: 13926–13931.

19. Gréen, K., Drvota, V., and Vesterqvist, O. Pronounced reduction of in vivo prostacyclin synthesis in humans by acetaminophen (paracetamol). *Prostaglandins* 1989; 37: 311–315.

20. Ridker, P.M., Rifai, N., Rose, L., Buring, J.E., and Cook, N.R. Comparison of C-reactive protein and low-density lipoprotein cholesterol levels in the prediction of first cardiovascular events. *N. Engl. J. Med.* 2002; 247: 1557–1565.

21. Shah, V.P., Midha, K.K., Findlay, J.W.A., Hill, H.M., Hulse, J.D., McGilvary, I.J., McKay, G., Miller, K.J., Patnaik, R.N., Powell, M.L., Tonnelli, A., Viswanathan, C.T., and Yacobi, A. Bioanalytical method validation: a revisit with a decade of progress. *Pharm Res.* 2000; 12: 1551–1557.

22. DeSilva, B., Smith, W., Wiener, R., Kelley, M., Smolec, J., Lee, B., Khan, M., Tacey, R., Hill, H., and Celniker, A. Recommendations for the bioanalytical method validation of ligand-binding assays to support pharmacokinetic assessments of macromolecules. *Pharm Res.* 2003; 20: 1885–1900.

23. Wadhwa, M., and Thorpe, R. Cytokine immunoassays: recommendations for standardisation, calibration and validation. *J. Immunol. Meth.* 1998; 219: 1–5.

24. Owens, M.A., Vall, H.G., Hurley, A.A., and Wormsley, S.B. Validation and quality control of immunophenotyping in clinical flow cytometry. *J. Immunol. Meth.* 2000; 243: 33–50.

25. Food and Drug Administration, Guidance for Industry, Exposure-Response Relationship: Study Design, Data Analysis, and Regulatory Applications. U.S. Dept. of Health and Human Services, Food and Drug Administration, April 2003.

26. Food and Drug Administration, Guidance for Industry, Bioanalytical Method Validation. U.S. Dept. of Health and Human Services, Food and Drug Administration, May 2001.

27. ICH Harmonised Tripartite Guideline. Validation of analytical procedures: *Methodology* 1996, November 6.

28. Westgard, J.O., and Klee, G.G. Quality management. In: Burtis, C.A., and Ashwood, E.R., Eds. *Tietz Textbook of Clinical Chemistry*, 3rd ed. Philadelphia: W.B. Saunders Co., 1999, 384–418.

29. Okegawa, T., Noda, H., Nutahara, K., and Higashihara, E. Comparison of two investigative assays for the complexed prostate-specific antigen in total prostate-specific antigen between 4.1 and 10.0 ng/mL. *Urology* 2000; 55: 700–704.

30. Juillerat, L., Nussberger, J., Menard, J., Mooser, V., Christen, Y., Waeber, B., Graf, P., and Brunner, H.R. Determinants of angiotensin II generation during converting enzyme inhibition. *Hypertension* 1990; 16: 564–572.

31. Vesterqvist, O., and Reeves, R.A. Effects of omapatrilat on pharmacodynamic biomarkers of neutral endopeptidase and angiotensin-converting enzyme activity in humans. *Curr. Hypertens. Rep.* 2001; 3(Suppl. 2): 22–27.

32. Food and Drug Administration, Challenge and Opportunity on the Critical Path to New Medical Products. U.S. Department of Health and Human Services, Food and Drug Administration, March 2004.

4 Opportunities in CNS Drug Discovery and Development

*Albert Pinhasov, Anil H. Vaidya, Hong Xin,
Daniel Horowitz, Daniel Rosenthal,
Douglas E. Brenneman, Ewa Malatynska,
Sergey E. Ilyin, and Carlos R. Plata-Salamán*

CONTENTS

Historically, the development of animal models for psychiatric disorders such as schizophrenia, anxiety, and depression has proven to be a challenging task. Indeed, it is difficult to ascertain the level of predictability or validation of an animal model to the human clinical condition. The development of animal models for psychiatric disorders was promoted after the introduction of chlorpromazine for the treatment of schizophrenia in 1954, and again after the introduction of chlordiazepoxide and valium for the treatment of anxiety in the 1960s. These turning points, along with the development of behavioral testing technology in experimental psychology after Skinner's publication of *Behavior of Organisms* in 1938, essentially brought into context the fields of psychology and pharmacology, leading to the emergence of the field of psychopharmacology (Carlton, 1983).

Drug discovery and drug development are long and complex processes within the pharmaceutical industry. Animal models continue to play an important role in this industry for screening drugs or for fully characterizing new molecular entities (NMEs) in the drug discovery stage, as they provide vital information that helps to determine whether an NME is actually useful in the clinic. Based on evaluation of drugs already known to have efficacy in humans for various psychiatric conditions, animal models have been undergoing continual refinement, and newer paradigms are being developed and validated for enhanced sophistication in terms of behavioral and therapeutic specificity.

The proposed predictive validity of animal models has led to their successful implementation in the pharmaceutical industry and, over the years, has resulted in an increasing trend of using behavioral models to screen compounds for efficacy and side-effects/toxicology. Furthermore, the sophistication and advancements in behavioral testing, such as telemetry, implementation of infrared-photocell technology, and digital video-tracking technology (which precisely tracks the movement of an animal in the testing apparatus), have provided the operational means for high-throughput *in vivo* testing. A combination of several of these methodologies also allows a fine analysis of behavioral specificity (e.g., whether a change in movement is due to specific changes of locomotor activity or to effects on motor coordination and balance, stereotypies, sedation, etc.).

Instrument and methodological advances can now be integrated with insights into behavioral testing and complementary approaches, i.e., testing in various models that provide combined know-how in an effort to collect as much relevant information as feasible considering the multiplicity, heterogeneity, and complex pathophysiology of neuropsychiatric manifestations and disorders. At the same time, refinement in behavioral testing also aids in the determination of specific and nonspecific behavioral effects, depending on the purpose as well as on the microstructure and domain analyses of a behavior via quantitative measures collected in real time by computerized behavioral monitoring systems and standardized methodologies and protocols. This approach can assist in reliability, replicability, and phenotype validation, especially when considering specific domains or segments of a behavior that may be associated with the induction or progression of a pathophysiological condition or response to a therapeutic intervention. Consistency of a specific behavioral profile across models and species, in the right setting and with appropriate interpretation, could build toward validation and understanding of complex behaviors. Overall, automation of behavioral testing has not only increased reliability and throughput of evaluating drugs *in vivo* for efficacy and safety in the preclinical stage, but has also prompted the refinement and integration of the data analysis process.

This chapter reviews various novel technologies and approaches currently used in drug discovery at the Johnson & Johnson Pharmaceutical Research and Development, LLC. These approaches range from automation of behavioral testing in a recently proposed model of depression, to the search and identification of biomarkers to substantiate models, to the use of high-throughput screening (HTS) robotics, and to the recently proposed novel paradigm for drug discovery known as *functional informatics*.

Researchers make every effort to automate behavioral tests in the neurosciences to minimize subjective judgment and manual labor and to maximize repeatability of the results between laboratories while increasing the throughput of experimental end points. In recent years, these efforts have accelerated due to (a) the development of many inbred or transgenic mice strains that needed systematic behavioral phenotyping to find the functions delineated to strain differences or specific genes, and (b) the development of *in vitro* biochemical high-throughput drug-screening tests, which highlighted similar needs in behavioral neurosciences where the intact organism is a subject of the study. The main concerns of adapting any behavioral test to large-scale screening of either drugs or animal strains include the reproducibility of measurement end points between laboratories; the throughput or capacity of the test; and, importantly, the validity of the test as a surrogate marker for human disease.

The problem of the reproducibility of measurement end points arose when some of the first transgenic animals were screened by similar behavioral methods, producing different and sometimes opposite behavioral results by independent laboratories (Crabbe et al., 1999). As a consequence, the standardization of behavioral tests was proposed, and several test batteries were developed (Crawley, 1999; Crawley and Paylor, 1997; Rogers et al., 1999; Tarantino et al., 2000).

Another approach to overcome differences in the interpretation of behavioral results between laboratories and to facilitate automatic analysis was a proposal to analyze a given behavior as a group of segments. As it is clearly understood, any behavioral response is more complex than a biochemical reaction because it emerges from the organism as a whole and involves multiple parallel and sequential biochemical and physiological pathways. However, even a relatively simple behavior such as locomotor activity is highly structured and consists of several patterns of exploratory or goal-oriented behaviors that can be further subdivided into episodes such as stops and progression segments (Kafkafi, 2003), each involving multiple neural pathways. Software for the exploration of exploration (SEE) was developed using this principle (Drai and Golani, 2001; Kafkafi, 2003). This software can characterize differences between distinct mouse strains in a highly structured manner using mathematical algorithms to analyze subtle patterns in mouse locomotor activity (Kafkafi, 2003).

The approach to solve the problem of test capacity while retaining the validity of the test as a surrogate marker for human disease is exemplified in the development of the "cat walk" test (Hamers et al., 2001; Vrinten and Hamers, 2003). Before the development of this method, mechanical allodynia was assessed by the stimulation of inflamed tissue with a series of von Fray filaments and observation of the withdrawal reaction (Chaplan et al., 1994). Responses were not always clear with this method and were very much observer dependent. The "cat walk" is an automated, computer-based gait-analysis method that enables objective and rapid quantification of several gait parameters such as different phases of the step cycle and the pressure applied during locomotion. With this method, it is possible to distinguish between spinal cord injuries and neuropathic pain expressed as mechanical allodynia (Hamers et al., 2001; Vrinten and Hamers, 2003).

The dominant–submissive reaction model is another approach which was designed to overcome problems of measurement precision and capacity while retaining relative value as a marker for the human condition of depression. Dominance and submissiveness, defined in a competition test and measured as the relative success of two food-restricted rats to gain access to a feeder, form a behavioral paradigm called the dominant–submissive relationship (DSR). This paradigm results in two models sensitive to drugs used to treat mood disorders. Drugs used to treat mania inhibit the dominant behavior of rats taking food at the expense of an opponent (reduction of dominant-behavior model, or RDBM). Antidepressant treatment increases the competitive behavior of submissive rats that lose in such encounters before treatment (reduction of submissive-behavior model, or RSBM). The RSBM belongs to a broader group of tests employed to study antidepressants that are based on social interactions of animals. They can be divided into three groups that measure the same main process — the ability of some animals to be superior (dominant) to others and the acceptance of others to be inferior (submissive) — in different ways. One group consists of the dominant–submissive interactions seen in groups of animals and measured mainly by observation of agonistic and defensive postures used to rank each animal's position in the group (Blanchard et al., 1987; Blanchard and Riley, 1988; Grant and Mackintosh, 1963; Mackintosh and Grant, 1966; Miczek and Barry, 1977). Another is represented by resident–intruder interactions, based on animal territoriality, that result in a defeated state that resembles aspects of depression (Kudryavtseva et al., 1991; Mitchell and Fletcher, 1993; Willner, 1995). A third group consists of winner–loser relations established in competition tests that measure priority of access to a desired resource (Malatynska et al., 2002; Malatynska and Kostowski, 1984; Masur and Benedito, 1974; Masur et al., 1971; Uyeno, 1966; Uyeno, 1967). The complexity of submissive and dominant social behaviors often results in controversy about their precise definition.

Previous efforts to measure dominant–submissive relationships have used descriptive rating scales that are difficult to share among laboratories (Kudryavtseva et al., 1991; Willner, 1995). Observed differences in specific submissive behaviors between mouse strains (Kudryavtseva et al., 1991) would complicate interstrain comparisons using such end points. This problem is addressed in the DSR, for example, by using the simple end point of milk drinking by competing animals. This is facilitated by the apparatus, which allows only one animal to consume milk at a time. Submissive behavior is measured as the relative difference in time spent drinking milk during a 5-minute interval between the dominant and submissive members of paired animals. This end point is unambiguous and eliminates inter-observer variability.

The precision of measuring DS behavior is also improved by the criteria applied to pair selection for having a dominant–submissive relationship. A pair is defined as having a dominant–submissive relation when: (a) the difference in time spent on the feeder by each animal from the pair is significantly different (P < .05) by the two-tail t test; (b) the difference in time spent on the feeder by each animal from the pair is 40% or more of the score value for the higher scoring (dominant) animal; and (c) there is no reversal of daily success as expressed by longer and shorter time spent on the feeder by an animal from the pair during the second week of observation time. Dominance measured by this behavioral procedure is a robust effect that is easily distinguished from submissiveness without complex subjective observations.

We have applied a multiple-subject video-tracking system (PanLab Software, San Diego Instruments, CA) to this method that automatically scores time spent by rats at the feeder (Pinhasov et al., 2005a). Using this method, it is possible to observe four pairs of rats during each 5-minute experimental session (one set). We have also used a duplicate parallel set with a second camera that enables immediate switch to the observation of the next four animals, thereby minimizing total experimental time. The multiple video-tracking systems reduced the variability between observations and improved throughput of dominant–submissive pairs by fivefold without increasing labor input. Thus, the number of animals available for drug testing is increased.

In summary, the automation of behavioral testing is a necessary next step in constructing precisely defined CNS diseases and pathophysiology models that will be repeatable between laboratories. The delineation of the model to a certain disease may improve with the segmentation of the given behavior and automatic parallel analysis of individual segments, domains, and subdomains. This would also serve to eliminate subjective scoring by observers. An application of this process was demonstrated in the SEE software and in the "cat walk" model. The requirement for model automation described above is also directly connected to the requirement for precise quantitative measurement, which was demonstrated in the DSR test by introducing a binary (positive or negative) end point. The process of automation of behavioral tests has only just started, and it is far behind the automation level of *in vitro* drug screening. However, it is possible that, with further understanding of the components of a complex behavior and with future technology improvements, its throughput will no longer be a serious limitation.

Behavioral pharmacology is an integral part of drug discovery and is essential for evaluation of drug activity. However, drug administration can activate labile and indirect mechanisms and thus mislead in the interpretation of effects caused by a drug. To address this question, the use of molecular biomarkers becomes a valuable addition for the evaluation of the mechanism of drug action. Furthermore, a better understanding of the molecular changes associated with the onset and progression of disease or of the temporal responses to drug administration provides a rational basis for the development of new diagnostic and therapeutic tools. For example, molecular markers such as beta-amyloid, prion protein (PrP), tau protein, and alpha-synuclein, which are basic components of specific brain lesions (amyloid plaques, prion plaques, tangles, and Lewy bodies, respectively), have dramatically improved the characterization and classification of numerous neurodegenerative diseases. In Alzheimer's disease, for example, phosphorylated tau and beta-amyloid deposition were prudently considered to be diagnostic markers (Hampel et al., 2003; Lewczuk et al., 2004; Nordberg, 2004). Discovery of molecular biomarkers also leads to the development of animal models, for example transgenic animals with overdeposition of beta-amyloid (Games et al., 1995; Hsiao et al., 1996) or with accumulation of phosphorylated tau (Gotz et al., 1995; Oddo et al., 2003a; Oddo et al., 2003b). Animal models can serve as a tool for revealing molecular biomarkers that can indicate whether certain alterations in physiological pathways will lead to patho-physiological cascades and disease.

We recently showed an example of such an approach by using the dominant–submissive relationship model for mania and depression (Malatynska et al., 2002), which was described above. In a more recent work using TaqMan quantitative reverse-transcriptase–polymerase chain reaction (RT-PCR) analysis (Pinhasov et al., 2004), it has been found that gamma-synuclein mRNA levels were down-regulated in the cerebral cortex of submissive rats (Pinhasov et al., 2005b). Hence, differential expression of gamma-synuclein in this model may provide initial insights into an aspect of the underlying pathophysiology in this condition and could provide novel tools for the development of new therapeutic interventions.

The development of microarray technologies (a) provides the advantage of being able to investigate the expression of thousands of genes simultaneously in treated versus control samples and (b) brings broader approaches to target identification (Palfreyman, 2002; Palfreyman et al., 2002). By using a microarray-based approach, one can compare normal and diseased tissue to obtain a "disease-associated profile or signature" of abnormally expressed genes. This is important, as the nature of neurological diseases is largely polygenic and can involve alteration in several biological pathways. Altar and colleagues studied the effects of electroconvulsive shock (ECS) exposures on gene transcription and identified genes that seem to be associated with the efficacy of chronic electroconvulsive therapy (ECT) (Altar et al., 2004) and found a complex pattern of differential gene expression among the treated and untreated subjects. Such a strategy could be used to identify lead compounds (Palfreyman, 2002; Palfreyman et al., 2002) that mimic the therapeutic response of ECT. Using the same approach, Altar et al. (2004) also investigated the effect of valproic acid on gene expression profiles of human postmortem parietal and prefrontal cortex samples of normal controls and of patients with bipolar disease; they ultimately identified a group of genes that was proposed to be associated with the disease condition. Overall, gene expression profiles can generate unique molecular patterns that direct to specific physiological–biochemical signaling systems associated with disease pathophysiology or cellular responses to drug administration.

Applications of molecular biomarkers can also translate to the use of diverse imaging methods such as single-photon emission computed tomography (SPECT), positron emission tomography (PET), and magnetic resonance imaging (MRI) (Marek and Seibyl, 2000). The combination of these methods with selective markers for various diseases can substantially impact the diagnosis and treatment of neurodegenerative diseases and also brings new perspectives in finding new drugs and other therapeutic interventions (Klunk et al., 2003). Direct *in vivo* detection of amyloid deposits in patients diagnosed with Alzheimer's disease and in the brains of transgenic animals of amyloid deposition using brain neuroimaging techniques would be well suited for the early diagnosis of Alzheimer's disease and the development and assessment of new treatment strategies (Nordberg, 2004; Okamura et al., 2004; Suemoto et al., 2004). MRI, which provides views of anatomic or structural brain abnormalities, has also been especially useful for assessing macroscopic neuromorphological changes in stroke and multiple sclerosis (Baird and Warach, 1999).

Drug administration associated with neuroactivity often involves alteration in neurotransmitter release (Adell and Artigas, 1998). Monitoring of neurotransmitter release is possible through the use of microdialysis methodology. The present pharmacotherapy of depression includes enhancement of central monoaminergic neurotransmission (Blier, 2003), and microdialysis is useful in the investigation of the effects of antidepressant agents on chemical neurotransmission, including in the synapsis (Adell and Artigas, 1998). Analysis and monitoring of acetylcholinergic mechanisms in cognitive and transgenic models of Alzheimer's disease also aid in the investigation of potential novel treatment strategies (Hartmann et al., 2004), and the assessment of amyloid-beta peptide in the brain interstitial fluid may offer new insights into amyloid-beta metabolism (Cirrito et al., 2003).

Combinations of different complementary drug-discovery approaches, such as behavioral pharmacology, genomics, and proteomics with molecular imaging and microdialysis, open new perspectives for the discovery of new molecular biomarkers. These integrated approaches to CNS drug discovery also increase the required tests that need to be conducted in concert with automated sample processing and analysis.

An interesting trend in the development of lab automation is that it comes out of a traditional HTS environment and then spreads to all areas of drug discovery and development. Its applications include, but are not limited to, early ADME (absorption, distribution, metabolism, and excretion) and toxicology studies, high-throughput proteomics, high-throughput target validation, and high-throughput biomarker discovery and validation. Instead of fully integrated systems, applications in these areas tend to rely more on integrated-workstation approaches. High-through-put target validation is a combination of traditional molecular biology methodologies with automation. Some examples are the small interfering RNA (siRNA)-based (Xin et al., 2004) and antisense-based approaches in combination with high-content screening. For high-throughput siRNA-based target validation, a fully integrated automation system for HTS was used to take full advantage of existing automation hardware (Xin et al., 2004). The assay has high throughput (2400 siRNAs could be tested in an 8-hour working day by one full-time employee) and great precision. The siRNA plates were tracked by the automation system, and data could be processed and queried automatically using a corporate database. This represents an example of an approach that allows large-scale siRNA-based target validation studies to be conducted in days rather than months, consequently reducing the timeline between target proposal and lead generation.

REFERENCES

Adell, A., and Artigas, F. (1998). A microdialysis study of the in vivo release of 5-HT in the median raphe nucleus of the rat. *Br. J. Pharmacol.* **125**, 1361–7.

Altar, C. A., Laeng, P., Jurata, L. W., Brockman, J. A., Lemire, A., Bullard, J., Bukhman, Y. V., Young, T. A., Charles, V., and Palfreyman, M. G. (2004). Electroconvulsive seizures regulate gene expression of distinct neurotrophic signaling pathways. *J. Neurosci.* **24**, 2667–77.

Baird, A. E., and Warach, S. (1999). Imaging developing brain infarction. *Curr. Opin. Neurol.* **12**, 65–71.

Blanchard, B. A., Hannigan, J. H., and Riley, E. P. (1987). Amphetamine-induced activity after fetal alcohol exposure and undernutrition in rats. *Neurotoxicol. Teratol.* **9**, 113–9.

Blanchard, B. A., and Riley, E. P. (1988). Effects of physostigmine on shuttle avoidance in rats exposed prenatally to ethanol. *Alcohol* **5**, 27–31.

Blier, P. (2003). The pharmacology of putative early-onset antidepressant strategies. *Eur. Neuropsychopharmacol.* **13**, 57–66.

Carlton, P. L. (1983). *A Primer of Behavioral Pharmacology: Concepts and Principles in the Behavioral Analysis of Drug Action.* W. H. Freeman, New York.

Chaplan, S. R., Bach, F. W., Pogrel, J. W., Chung, J. M., and Yaksh, T. L. (1994). Quantitative assessment of tactile allodynia in the rat paw. *J. Neurosci. Methods* **53**, 55–63.

Cirrito, J. R., May, P. C., O'Dell, M. A., Taylor, J. W., Parsadanian, M., Cramer, J. W., Audia, J. E., Nissen, J. S., Bales, K. R., Paul, S. M., DeMattos, R. B., and Holtzman, D. M. (2003). In vivo assessment of brain interstitial fluid with microdialysis reveals plaque-associated changes in amyloid-beta metabolism and half-life. *J. Neurosci.* **23**, 8844–53.

Crabbe, J. C., Wahlsten, D., and Dudek, B. C. (1999). Genetics of mouse behavior: interactions with laboratory environment [see comments]. *Science* **284**, 1670–2.

Crawley, J. N. (1999). Behavioral phenotyping of transgenic and knockout mice: experimental design and evaluation of general health, sensory functions, motor abilities, and specific behavioral tests. *Brain Res.* **835**, 18–26.

Crawley, J. N., and Paylor, R. (1997). A proposed test battery and constellations of specific behavioral paradigms to investigate the behavioral phenotypes of transgenic and knockout mice. *Horm. Behav.* **31**, 197–211.

Drai, D., and Golani, I. (2001). SEE: a tool for the visualization and analysis of rodent exploratory behavior. *Neurosci. Biobehav. Rev.* **25**, 409–26.

Games, D., Adams, D., Alessandrini, R., Barbour, R., Berthelette, P., Blackwell, C., Carr, T., Clemens, J., Donaldson, T., Gillespie, F., et al. (1995). Alzheimer-type neuropathology in transgenic mice overexpressing V717F beta-amyloid precursor protein. *Nature* **373**, 523–7.

Gotz, J., Probst, A., Spillantini, M. G., Schafer, T., Jakes, R., Burki, K., and Goedert, M. (1995). Somatodendritic localization and hyperphosphorylation of tau protein in transgenic mice expressing the longest human brain tau isoform. *EMBO J.* **14**, 1304–13.

Grant, E. C., and Mackintosh, J. H. (1963). A comparison of the social postures of some common laboratory rodents. *Behaviour* **21**, 246–59.

Hamers, F. P., Lankhorst, A. J., van Laar, T. J., Veldhuis, W. B., and Gispen, W. H. (2001). Automated quantitative gait analysis during overground locomotion in the rat: its application to spinal cord contusion and transection injuries. *J. Neurotrauma* **18**, 187–201.

Hampel, H., Goernitz, A., and Buerger, K. (2003). Advances in the development of biomarkers for Alzheimer's disease: from CSF total tau and Abeta(1-42) proteins to phosphorylated tau protein. *Brain. Res. Bull.* **61**, 243–53.

Hartmann, J., Erb, C., Ebert, U., Baumann, K. H., Popp, A., Konig, G., and Klein, J. (2004). Central cholinergic functions in human amyloid precursor protein knock-in/presenilin-1 transgenic mice. *Neuroscience* **125**, 1009–17.

Hsiao, K., Chapman, P., Nilsen, S., Eckman, C., Harigaya, Y., Younkin, S., Yang, F., and Cole, G. (1996). Correlative memory deficits, Abeta elevation, and amyloid plaques in transgenic mice. *Science* **274**, 99–102.

Kafkafi, N. (2003). Extending SEE for large-scale phenotyping of mouse open-field behavior. *Behav. Res. Methods Instrum. Comput.* **35**, 294–301.

Klunk, W. E., Engler, H., Nordberg, A., Bacskai, B. J., Wang, Y., Price, J. C., Bergstrom, M., Hyman, B. T., Langstrom, B., and Mathis, C. A. (2003). Imaging the pathology of Alzheimer's disease: amyloid-imaging with positron emission tomography. *Neuroimaging Clin. N. Am.* **13**, 781–9, ix.

Kudryavtseva, N. N., Bakshtanovskaya, I. V., and Koryakina, L. A. (1991). Social model of depression in mice of C57BL/6J strain. *Pharmacol. Biochem. Behav.* **38**, 315–20.

Lewczuk, P., Esselmann, H., Bibl, M., Beck, G., Maler, J. M., Otto, M., Kornhuber, J., and Wiltfang, J. (2004). Tau protein phosphorylated at threonine 181 in CSF as a neurochemical biomarker in Alzheimer's disease: original data and review of the literature. *J. Mol. Neurosci.* **23**, 115–22.

Mackintosh, J. H., and Grant, E. C. (1966). The effect of olfactory stimuli on the agonistic behaviour of laboratory mice. *Z. Tierpsychol.* **23**, 584–7.

Malatynska, E., Goldenberg, R., Shuck, L., Haque, A., Zamecki, P., Crites, G., Schindler, N., and Knapp, R. J. (2002). Reduction of submissive behavior in rats: a test for antidepressant drug activity. *Pharmacology* **64**, 8–17.

Malatynska, E., and Kostowski, W. (1984). The effect of antidepressant drugs on dominance behavior in rats competing for food. *Pol. J. Pharmacol. Pharm.* **36**, 531–40.

Marek, K., and Seibyl, J. (2000). TechSight. Imaging. A molecular map for neurodegeneration. *Science* **289**, 409–11.

Masur, J., and Benedito, M. A. (1974). Genetic selection of winner and loser rats in a competitive situation. *Nature* **249**, 284.

Masur, J., Martz, R. M., Bieniek, D., and Korte, F. (1971). Influence of (−) 9-trans-tetrahydrocannabinol and mescaline on the behavior of rats submitted to food competition situations. *Psychopharmacologia* **22**, 187–94.

Miczek, K. A., and Barry, H., III (1977). Effects of alcohol on attack and defensive-submissive reactions in rats. *Psychopharmacology (Berl.)* **52**, 231–7.

Mitchell, P. J., and Fletcher, A. (1993). Venlafaxine exhibits pre-clinical antidepressant activity in the resident-intruder social interaction paradigm. *Neuropharmacology* **32**, 1001–9.

Nordberg, A. (2004). PET imaging of amyloid in Alzheimer's disease. *Lancet Neurol.* **3**, 519–27.

Oddo, S., Caccamo, A., Kitazawa, M., Tseng, B. P., and LaFerla, F. M. (2003a). Amyloid deposition precedes tangle formation in a triple transgenic model of Alzheimer's disease. *Neurobiol. Aging* **24**, 1063–70.

Oddo, S., Caccamo, A., Shepherd, J. D., Murphy, M. P., Golde, T. E., Kayed, R., Metherate, R., Mattson, M. P., Akbari, Y., and LaFerla, F. M. (2003b). Triple-transgenic model of Alzheimer's disease with plaques and tangles: intracellular Abeta and synaptic dysfunction. *Neuron* **39**, 409–21.

Okamura, N., Suemoto, T., Shiomitsu, T., Suzuki, M., Shimadzu, H., Akatsu, H., Yamamoto, T., Arai, H., Sasaki, H., Yanai, K., Staufenbiel, M., Kudo, Y., and Sawada, T. (2004). A novel imaging probe for in vivo detection of neuritic and diffuse amyloid plaques in the brain. *J Mol. Neurosci.* **24**, 247–56.

Palfreyman, M. G. (2002). Human tissue in target identification and drug discovery. *Drug Discov. Today* **7**, 407–9.

Palfreyman, M. G., Hook, D. J., Klimczak, L. J., Brockman, J. A., Evans, D. M., and Altar, C. A. (2002). Novel directions in antipsychotic target identification using gene arrays. *Curr. Drug Targets CNS Neurol. Disord.* **1**, 227–38.

Pinhasov, A., Crooke, J., Rosenthal, D., Brenneman, D., and Malatynska, E. (2005a). Reduction of submissive behavior model for antidepressant drug activity testing: study using a video-tracking system. *Behav. Pharmacol.* **16**, 657–64.

Pinhasov, A., Ilyin, S. E., Crooke, J., Amato, F. A., Vaidya, A. H., Rosenthal, D., Brenneman, D. E., and Malatynska, E. (2005b). Different levels of gamma-synuclein mRNA in the cerebral cortex of dominant, neutral and submissive rats selected in the competition test. *Genes Brain Behav.* **4**, 60–4.

Pinhasov, A., Mei, J., Amaratunga, D., Amato, F. A., Lu, H., Kauffman, J., Xin, H., Brenneman, D. E., Johnson, D. L., Andrade-Gordon, P., and Ilyin, S. E. (2004). Gene expression analysis for high throughput screening applications. *Comb. Chem. High Throughput Screen* **7**, 133–40.

Rogers, D. C., Jones, D. N., Nelson, P. R., Jones, C. M., Quilter, C. A., Robinson, T. L., and Hagan, J. J. (1999). Use of SHIRPA and discriminant analysis to characterise marked differences in the behavioural phenotype of six inbred mouse strains. *Behav. Brain Res.* **105**, 207–17.

Suemoto, T., Okamura, N., Shiomitsu, T., Suzuki, M., Shimadzu, H., Akatsu, H., Yamamoto, T., Kudo, Y., and Sawada, T. (2004). In vivo labeling of amyloid with BF-108. *Neurosci. Res.* **48**, 65–74.

Tarantino, L. M., Gould, T. J., Druhan, J. P., and Bucan, M. (2000). Behavior and mutagenesis screens: the importance of baseline analysis of inbred strains. *Mamm. Genome* **11**, 555–64.

Uyeno, E. T. (1966). Effects of D-lysergic acid diethylamide and 2-brom-lysergic acid diethyl-amide on dominance behavior of the rat. *Int. J. Neuropharmacol.* **5**, 317–22.

Uyeno, E. T. (1967). Effects of mescaline and psilocybin on dominance behavior of the rat. *Arch. Int. Pharmacodyn. Ther.* **166**, 60–4.

Vrinten, D. H., and Hamers, F. F. (2003). "CatWalk" automated quantitative gait analysis as a novel method to assess mechanical allodynia in the rat; a comparison with von Frey testing. *Pain* **102**, 203–9.

Willner, P. (1995). Animal models of depression: validity and applications. *Adv. Biochem. Psychopharmacol.* **49**, 19–41.

Xin, H., Bernal, A., Amato, F. A., Pinhasov, A., Kauffman, J., Brenneman, D. E., Derian, C. K., Andrade-Gordon, P., Plata-Salaman, C. R., and Ilyin, S. E. (2004). High-throughput siRNA-based functional target validation. *J. Biomol. Screen* **9**, 286–93.

5 Clinical Success of Antibody Therapeutics in Oncology

Bernard J. Scallon, Linda A. Snyder,
G. Mark Anderson, Qiming Chen, Li Yan,
and Marian T. Nakada

CONTENTS

INTRODUCTION

The antibodies currently approved for the treatment of diseases, including cancer, have been developed predominantly based on the understanding and identification of key targets involved in disease pathology. Thus, for oncology, currently marketed antibodies to epidermal growth-factor receptors/human epidermal growth-factor receptor (EGFR/HER1 and HER2) and vascular endothelial growth factor (VEGF) treat cancer by blocking the function of these targets that are crucial for tumor progression. Other targets for launched products are those that are highly upregulated on neoplastic cells, including CD20, CD52, and CD33. Antibodies are generally highly specific for their molecular targets and can be used to affect disease-specific targets, thereby sparing normal cells and causing less toxicity than traditional cytotoxic chemotherapies. Effective antibodies act through one or more of a variety of mechanisms, including (a) blocking essential cellular growth factors or receptors; (b) directly inducing apoptosis; (c) binding to target cells and recruiting "effector functions," such as antibody-dependent cellular cytotoxicity (ADCC) or complement-dependent cytotoxicity (CDC); and (d) delivering cytotoxic payloads such as chemotherapies, radioisotopes, and toxins.

The use of informatics will be essential as we develop new waves of products that provide additional efficacy, specificity, or safety over currently marketed products. Informatics approaches can be used to (a) identify novel targets either upstream or downstream of already validated targets to enhance or complement efficacy; (b) identify targets that are more specific for tumors, thereby enhancing safety and providing a means of directing toxic agents to the tumor; (c) identify novel pathways essential for disease progression; and (d) identify Fc mutants that have enhanced immune-effector function. The sections below describe the current state of antibody technology and drug development for oncology and suggest how informatics is providing valuable tools to advance these efforts.

ANTIBODY TECHNOLOGY

The first monoclonal antibodies from mice were generated in 1975 [1]. In humans, mouse-derived antibodies are highly immunogenic, and therefore "chimeric" antibodies were created by replacing mouse-constant domains (nonantigen-binding domains) with human-constant domains [2]. This improvement considerably reduced the immune response to therapeutic antibodies. Additional modifications of framework regions within the antigen-binding variable regions further reduced immunogenicity, resulting in what is termed "humanized" antibodies. Fully human antibodies can be derived from human cells or from genetically engineered mice that are transgenic for human antibody genes. Human antibodies can also be generated from antibody-expressing phage libraries as single-chain Fv or Fab fragments that can subsequently be converted to full-length antibodies [2].

ANTIBODIES THAT ARE APPROVED AND IN LATE-STAGE CLINICAL DEVELOPMENT

The promise of harnessing the power of antibodies to treat cancer is now being realized in clinical practice. There are currently eight FDA-approved monoclonal antibodies for oncology indications (Table 5.1) [3]. Most of the approved antibodies, and those in late-stage clinical trials, were designed to directly target antigens known to be expressed on tumor cells and, in some instances, known to mediate essential disease-critical functions. A majority of these targets are cell-surface receptors, most notably receptor tyrosine kinases that mediate signaling processes necessary for essential cellular functions and for maintaining the malignant phenotypes of tumor cells [4]. Other antibody drugs bind to antigens overexpressed on tumor cells and mediate their effects through antibody-effector function or the delivery of a toxic payload. The hope is that greater efficacy can be achieved by combining antibody therapy with chemotherapy, other biologics, or radiotherapy. Animal models using these antibodies have shown additive or synergistic benefits when combined with chemotherapy or other biologic therapies [5].

PROMISING ANTIBODIES AND TARGETS

The success in designing and developing antibody-based cancer therapy depends largely on selecting suitable targets. In general, monoclonal antibody targets need to meet the following criteria: (a) the target antigen is expressed by tumor cells at a much higher level than by normal cells; (b) the antigen must be presented properly and stably on the tumor cell surface for its recognition by the antibody; (c) the antigen is expressed by a large percentage of tumor cells, and is expressed in a broad spectrum of different types of tumor; and (d) the antigen functionally participates in the malignant disease process and, ideally, would be essential for multiple steps during such processes.

These selection criteria were well reflected by two recently approved antibody therapeutics for treating solid tumors, Avastin [6] and Erbitux [7]. Avastin, the anti-VEGF antibody, neutralizes the activity of VEGF, one of the most potent angiogenic growth factors. Erbitux, the anti-EGFR antibody, binds and blocks the signaling through the receptor tyrosine kinase. These two antibodies together with Herceptin highlight the antibody therapeutics against cell-surface receptors or associated signaling pathways.

A review of currently approved antibody therapeutics (Table 5.1) reveals another major category of tumor cell-surface antigens: various CD molecules. These cell-surface CD molecules — CD20, CD22, CD33, and CD52 — are overexpressed on tumor cells, most notably those of hematopoetic origin. Antibodies to these targets are being developed in the form of naked antibodies, antibody-conjugated toxin, or as radiolabeled antibodies.

Oncofetal proteins are expressed during fetal development, and then expression is partially or completely repressed in adult tissues. For some oncofetal proteins, expression is derepressed in some tissues that have undergone neoplastic transformation. Classical oncofetal antigens such as alpha-fetoprotein, CA125, carcinoembryonic antigen, and pancreatic oncofetal antigen are useful tumor markers. Antibodies to these and other oncofetal proteins such as Lewis X and Y, tumor-associated glycoprotein-72 (TAG-72), the early thymic antigen UN1, and oncofetal fibronectin are currently being evaluated.

In addition to targeting tumor cell-surface antigens, antibodies that target the tumor vasculature represent an attractive approach. Tumor growth is dependent on

TABLE 5.1
Oncology Antibodies Approved by the USFDA

Name (U.S. Trade Name)[a]	Company	Target	Mechanism	Antibody Form[b]	Cancer Indication	USFDA Approval Date	Ref.
Rituximab (Rituxan®)	Genentech and IDEC Pharmaceuticals	CD20	ADCC, CDC, directly induces apoptosis	Chimeric IgG1	NHL	11/97	[113]
Trastuzumab (Herceptin®)	Genentech	HER2	Inhibition of HER2-mediated tumor cell proliferation and migration	Humanized IgG1	Breast cancer with HER2 overexpression	9/98	[114]
Gemtuzumab ozogamicin (Mylotarg®)	Wyeth-Ayerst and Celltech Group	CD33	Delivery of calicheamicin into leukemic cells, resulting in DNA strand breaks and apoptosis	Humanized IgG4 linked to calicheamicin	AML	5/00	[115]
Alemtuzumab (Campath®)	Ilex Pharmaceuticals and Berlex Laboratories	CD52	ADCC, CDC	Humanized IgG1	CLL	5/01	[116]
Ibritumomab tiuxetan (Zevalin™)	IDEC Pharmaceuticals	CD20	Delivery of cytotoxic radiation, ADCC, CDC, apoptosis	Murine IgG1 ^{90}Y conjugate (murine parent form of rituximab) (Rituximab preceding Indium-111 Zevalin followed seven to nine days later by a second infusion of rituximab prior to Yttrium-90 Zevalin)	NHL	2/02	[117]

Tositumomab/ 131I-tositumomab (Bexxar®)	Corixia and GlaxoSmithKline	CD20	Delivery of cytotoxic radiation, ADCC, CDC, apoptosis	Murine IgG2a 131I conjugate plus unlabeled antibody	NHL	6/03	[118]
Bevacizumab (Avastin™)	Genentech	VEGF	Inhibition of VEGF-induced angiogenesis	Humanized IgG1	Metastatic colorectal cancer	2/04	[119]
Cetuximab (Erbitux™)	ImClone Systems and Bristol Myers Squibb	EGFR (HER1)	Inhibits EGFR-mediated tumor cell invasion, proliferation, and metastasis and angiogenesis Enhances activity of some chemotherapeutics and radiotherapy	Chimeric IgG1	Metastatic colorectal cancer	2/04	[120]

Note: ADCC – antibody-dependent cytotoxicity; CDC – complement-dependent cytotoxicity; NHL – non-Hodgkin's lymphoma; AML – acute myeloid leukemia; CLL – chronic lymphocytic leukemia; EGFR, HER1, HER2 – epidermal growth factor receptors; US – United States; FDA – Food and Drug Administration; VEGF – vascular endothelial growth factor.

[a] The suffixes of the generic names of antibodies are assigned as follows: murine antibodies are "omab," chimeric antibodies are "ximab," humanized antibodies are "zumab," and fully human antibodies are "umab."

[b] Human IgG1 and IgG2 isotypes are effective in inducing CDC and ADCC, whereas the IgG4 isotype is marginally effective for both. IgG2 has CDC activity but little to no ADCC activity.

angiogenesis, the formation of new blood vessels. Targeting tumor vessels provides several advantages over traditional antitumor approaches, including the genetic stability of antigen expression on tumor endothelial cells and the resulting low likelihood of developing drug resistance, broad application to various tumor types, and low toxicity to normal tissues [8]. The antiangiogenesis concept has been validated in clinical studies by the success of Avastin in treating metastatic colorectal cancer [7]. Antibodies have also been developed to endothelial cell-adhesion molecules, integrins (αVβ3/αVβ5 and α5β1), vascular endothelial (VE)-cadherin, occludin, E-selectin, and platelet/endothelial-specific cell-adhesion molecule (PECAM). In advanced development stage are antibodies against αVβ3 integrin, an antigen expressed on certain tumor cells and the surface of endothelial cells actively involved in tumor angiogenesis, but not of those lining quiescent blood vessels. Vitaxin™, a humanized antibody to αvβ3, and CNTO 95, a fully human monoclonal antibody to αVβ3/αVβ5, have successfully completed phase I clinical studies in patients with advanced cancer [9, 10].

Other targets that are suitable for monoclonal antibody-based anticancer therapeutics may derive from tumor stromal cells. The critical role of tumor stromal cells and tumor–host interactions is now becoming increasingly appreciated [11]. The composition, integrity, and the mechanical properties of the basement membrane have substantial influence on tumor cell behaviors, from tumor growth to metastasis. Enzymes of matrix metalloproteinase (MMP) and plasminogen activator (PA) (urokinase PA and tissue PA) systems are important players in remodeling the extracellular matrix (ECM), and in regulating the availability of biologically active ECM-bound growth factors. Despite the disappointing clinical trial results of small-molecule MMP inhibitors, the enzymes or proteins that modulate the activity of these enzymes remain attractive antibody targets. Interactions between tumor and host are also regulated by different soluble growth factors, cytokines, and chemokines. These inflammatory factors represent another group of potential targets [12]. For example, tumor necrosis factor α (TNFα) plays a crucial role in cancer progression, and blockade of TNFα with the chimeric antibody Remicade® (infliximab) has demonstrated promising therapeutic efficacy in treating metastatic renal cell cancer [13]. In addition to being therapeutics, these anti-inflammatory antibodies may also have the potential to provide supportive-care benefits [14].

SUPPORTIVE CARE

Advancements toward earlier detection and improved outcomes with new targeted therapies promise to transform cancer into a chronic and manageable condition rather than a uniformly fatal disease. In this context, ameliorating symptoms caused by the underlying cancer or side effects of toxic therapies with supportive care are increasingly important in the management and treatment of cancer. The advent of molecular biological and bioinformatic techniques makes it possible to begin to understand the pathological basis of cancer-associated cachexia, pain, and depression, for example. In addition to acting as tumor therapeutics, antibodies may be especially well suited to supportive care in treatment of cancer, given their targeted nature.

TNFα is a good example of a potential antibody target for supportive care in treatment of cancer, as TNFα is believed to play a crucial role in mediating cancer-related morbidity. The utility of blocking TNFα with the chimeric antibody Remicade is under preclinical and clinical investigation. Remicade is currently FDA-approved for the treatment of immune-mediated inflammatory disorders, including Crohn's disease and rheumatoid arthritis. The range of potential indications for supportive care is broad and diverse due to the pleiotropism of TNFα action and includes cancer-associated depression, fatigue, cachexia, treatment of toxicities due to chemotherapy and radiotherapy, treatment of metastatic bone pain, and graft versus host disease (GVHD) [15–19].

A wealth of evidence implicates TNFα as a mediator of cachexia [20]. In fact, TNFα was initially called "cachectin" because it caused severe wasting in rodent models of disease. TNFα has also been shown to be important for cachexia at the cellular and molecular levels, both by increasing destructive proteolysis in mature skeletal muscle and by inhibiting the differentiation of myoblasts necessary for the repair of damaged or stressed muscle tissue [21].The molecular details of TNFα action on skeletal muscle are starting to be elucidated. Acharyya et al. [22] provide evidence that TNFα, acting in concert with interferon γ (IFNγ), specifically down-regulates the expression of myosin heavy chain. These observations help to explain the molecular pathology of cancer-related cachexia and may point the way to measurable pharmacodynamic markers of anti-TNFα activity. Clinical trials are now testing the ability of anti-TNFα agents such as Remicade to inhibit wasting in cancer patients [20, 23]. Additional targets that have been associated with cancer cachexia and may be attractive antibody targets include interleukin (IL)-1, IL-6, proteolysis inducing factor (PIF), and IFNγ [23].

Several other cancer-associated conditions could be potentially attributed to TNFα activity. Cancer-related pain remains a significant unmet medical need. TNFα appears to be important both for the pain signal itself as well as metastatic bone erosion [24, 25]. TNFα also appears to mediate many of the unwanted side effects of radiation therapy. Radiation-induced production of TNFα by tumor cells enhances the intended local proinflammatory effects of ionizing radiation, but also damages normal tissue and can cause unwanted fibrosis. Preclinical and clinical data suggest that TNFα plays a role in mediating radiation-induced normal tissue damage and fibrosis and that anti-TNFα therapy may be effective treatment for the prevention of these deleterious side effects [26, 27].

NOVEL ANTIBODY TARGET DISCOVERY IN THE GENOMICS AND PROTEOMICS AGE

Recent advances in gene-expression analysis have enabled large-scale gene profiling to identify "tumor-specific" antigens. These techniques include serial analysis of gene expression (SAGE), reverse transcriptase–polymerase chain reaction (RT-PCR)-based differential display, subtractive hybridization, expressed sequence tag (EST) sequencing, and most importantly DNA microarray, all of which are used for detecting overexpressed genes, alternative splicing forms, mutations, and fusion transcripts that are specific to tumor cells. With the introduction of laser-captured microdissection and *in vitro* linear gene amplification, it has become feasible to compare the expression profile of virtually all human gene transcripts in cancerous cells versus their adjacent normal counterparts [28]. In addition to altered gene-expression levels, cancer cells also exhibit dysregulation in their protein synthesis and modification machineries. For example, changes in posttranslational modification are known to be responsible for unregulated cell growth and are implicated in tumorigenesis, representing yet another class of antibody targets. Therefore, it is also critical to analyze these changes in cancer cell proteins via proteomic approaches to identify novel cancer therapeutic targets [29].

Given the importance of cell-surface proteins as target antigens for therapeutic antibodies in treating cancer, it is obviously attractive to develop antibodies to tumor-specific antigens in a high-throughput fashion. With the complete human genome sequence unraveled, genes encoding cell-surface antigens could be reliably predicted by bioinformatic analysis. These selected genes could be cloned, synthesized, and expressed to serve as antigens. Alternatively, phage display presents another approach to generate such antibodies. Phages harboring antibody-encoding genes could be hybridized with tumor tissue sections. Phages bound to tumor cells and preferentially recognizing tumor-specific antigens can be retrieved to express such antibodies for further characterization in various tumor models. This "reverse immunology" approach could also be combined with proteomics technology in which monoclonal antibodies could be generated to proteins such as those derived from tumor cell membrane protein preparations that have been separated on two-dimensional gel electrophoresis [30]. Proteomics used in combination with antibody engineering also provides a means to generate such antibodies as Omnitarg™ (pertuzumab, 2C4), the new anti-HER2 antibody with a distinct mechanism of action to Herceptin [31]. Because Omnitarg binds to specific epitopes of HER2 receptor involved in HER2 heterodimerization with other HER receptors and sterically blocks signaling from these receptors, its anticancer activity is independent of high HER2 expression and could be applicable in multiple cancer types in addition to breast cancer [32]. Such approaches may be especially useful in designing and developing novel antibodies to cell-surface receptors such as tyrosine kinase receptor family members.

APPROACHES TO ENHANCING ANTIBODY EFFICACY

Enhancing Antibody Immune-Effector Functions

One of the more important activities of antibodies is to help trigger cellular immune responses against various targets, such as a pathogen, a pathogen-infected host cell, or a tumor cell. One way this is accomplished is for an antibody to bind to its cellular target via its antigen-binding Fab domains while simultaneously binding to IgG Fc receptors (FcγR) expressed on nearby immune-effector cells. Engagement of FcγRs on these effector cells, which can be macrophages, monocytes, dendritic cells, natural killer (NK) cells, or neutrophils, can lead them either to phagocytose the antibody-bound target, to kill the antibody-bound target by inducing ADCC, or to kill the target by releasing soluble lytic factors. Cellular immune responses can also be induced by antibodies via complement-dependent cell cytotoxicity (CDCC), in which components of the complement cascade serve to enhance or recruit the activity of cytotoxic effector cells. Another antibody-mediated immune-effector function related to CDCC that does not directly involve cellular responses is complement-dependent cytotoxicity (CDC), in which the thorough progression through the complement cascade results in formation of a cell-lysing membrane-attack complex on the antigen-expressing cell. Engineering of antibody molecules to be more effective at recruiting these functions has been of great interest, particularly for cancer immunotherapy. If successful, such efforts will lead to multiple benefits, including improved clinical efficacy, a greater proportion of treated patients responding to therapy, lower dosing, and reduced costs for treatment.

General Description of FcγRs

There are two main types of FcγRs on the surface of immune-effector cells when categorized by function: activating FcγRs and inhibiting FcγRs [33, 34]. Both types of FcγR bind IgG molecules in a 1:1 stoichiometric ratio in the region that spans the lower-hinge and upper-Fc domains. The activating FcγRs, which transmit pro-inflammatory types of signals upon IgG binding, are the high-affinity receptor, CD64 (FcγRI), and the low-affinity receptors, CD32A (FcγRIIA) and CD16A (FcγRIIIA). CD64 is the only FcγR that readily binds to monomeric IgG. It is expressed on monocytes, macrophages, and dendritic cells, and it can be induced to express on neutrophils by interferon-γ. CD32A and CD16A show minimal binding to monomeric IgG, but they show very significant binding to higher-order immune complexes of IgG due to the avidity effect associated with numerous hinge/Fc domains within a complex, simultaneously binding numerous FcγRs on a cell. CD32A is primarily expressed on monocytes, macrophages, dendritic cells, neutrophils, eosinophils, and platelets, whereas CD16A is primarily expressed on macrophages and NK cells. The inhibiting FcγR is CD32B (FcγRIIB), which can interrupt intracellular signaling events triggered by activating FcγRs on the same cell. CD32B is expressed on monocytes, macrophages, and B cells. The net cellular responses that result from binding of IgG immune complexes to FcγR on cells that express both activating and inhibiting FcRs probably depend on several factors, such as the relative expression level of the two types of FcγR, the relative avidity of the immune complexes to the different FcγRs present, and the relative "strength" of intracellular signaling pathways from the opposing FcγR types.

The molecular events that lead to FcγR binding and intracellular signaling were previously suspected to involve altered Fc conformations that distinguish antigen-bound antibodies from nonantigen-bound antibodies. However, it is now widely accepted that it is the clustering of the low-affinity FcγRs by multivalent antibody–antigen immune complexes that leads to intracellular signaling. The high-affinity FcγR, CD64, is constantly binding antibodies, whether the antibodies are bound to antigen or not. Such binding leads to receptor-mediated internalization of both receptor and antibody. However, the fate of such internalized antibodies is believed to depend on whether they are clustered by antigen. Antibodies that are not clustered, as well as the CD64 receptor itself, are thought to recycle back to the cell surface, whereas clustered antibodies (higher-order immune complexes) are retained in the cell and routed through a lysosome-mediated degradation pathway [35, 36]. What is not as clear is the fate of monovalent antigens bound to antibody in a simple 1:1 or 2:1 complex (i.e., where antibodies are not clustered) after binding and internalization of the complex through CD64.

Preclinical and Clinical Evidence for the Importance of FcγRs in Antibody Therapy

The importance of FcγRs to the antitumor activity of antibodies in a mouse model was neatly demonstrated using mice that lacked either the activating FcγRs or the inhibiting FcγR. Antitumor antibodies were less effective at controlling tumors in mice that lacked activating FcγRs compared with wild-type mice, but were substantially more effective in mice that lacked the inhibiting FcγR [37]. These data not only confirmed the contrasting roles of the activating and inhibiting FcγRs, but also helped inspire ongoing efforts to prepare novel antitumor antibodies that would favor binding to the activating FcγRs over the inhibiting FcγR.

Although it has been known for some time that different individuals have slightly different variations of particular FcγRs, the importance of such allotypic variants to clinical response to antibody therapy has only recently been appreciated. Cartron et al. [38] showed that non-Hodgkin lymphoma patients that were homozygous for a CD16A receptor that has a Val at position 158 had better clinical responses to rituximab (IgG1 antibody that binds CD20) than patients that were homozygous for a CD16A receptor that has a Phe at that position. Given that the Val^{158} allotype is known to bind IgG1 with higher affinity than the Phe^{158} allotype, such data was the first to convincingly implicate FcγR binding as an important part of the mechanism of action for a therapeutic antibody. A subsequent study that compared clinical responses to rituximab in follicular lymphoma patients that varied with respect to both CD16 and CD32 FcγR allotypes implicated both CD16 and CD32 FcγRs as playing a role in responses to rituximab [39]. Although there is evidence that higher antibody dosing could help to compensate for reduced binding to antibody in those patients with a lower-binding allotype of CD16 [40], the above findings helped prompt a further acceleration of efforts to enhance the FcγR-mediated effector functions of antibodies.

Choosing an IgG Isotype

Probably the earliest efforts to optimize the effector function of therapeutic antibodies were based on simply choosing the desired IgG isotype, wherein recombinant DNA methods were used to fuse the DNA encoding the heavy-chain variable-region portion of the antibody with DNA encoding the constant region (isotype) of either IgG1, IgG2, IgG3, or IgG4. The IgG1 isotype of human antibodies has long been the choice when immune-effector functions such as ADCC and CDC are desired. IgG3 antibodies also show high-affinity binding to FcγRs and are potent activators of CDC, but are problematic for commercial development owing to their propensity to self-associate and form aggregates. IgG1 may be the choice isotype even when immune-effector functions are not believed to be part of the mechanism of action for an antibody. This is because binding to either of the low-affinity FcγRs, as well as triggering of the classical complement pathway, requires a local cluster of antibodies, which may not ever form in the case of soluble antibody–antigen complexes that never expand beyond one antibody molecule binding to two antigen molecules. IgG4 antibodies are viewed by some as lacking immune-effector functions when, in fact, there are data that IgG4s are either just as active or perhaps only five- or tenfold less active than their IgG1 counterparts in FcγR-dependent activities [41, 42]. The variable assessments of how IgG4s compare with IgG1s in Fc-mediated activities can probably be attributed to the range of biological assays used, since there are indications that the difference between the two IgG isotypes ranges from substantial (in the case of low-affinity FcγR binding) to moderate (in the case of monomeric IgG binding to high-affinity CD64) to minimal or none (in the case of binding assays that involve a mix of cell types in which one expresses cell-surface antigen and the other expresses CD64 FcγR). The clear exception, however, appears to be *in vitro* CDC activity, in which IgG4s show very little or no activity but IgG1s are highly active.

Any decision to develop an IgG4 antibody should take into consideration the phenomenon of what could be called HL exchange between unrelated IgG4 molecules [43]. Although it has been known for many years that a significant proportion of the molecules in preparations of purified IgG4 monoclonal antibodies lacks disulfide bonds between the two heavy chains, only recently has it been shown that the two HL dimers of an $(HL)_2$ tetrameric IgG4 can dissociate from each other and then reassociate with an HL dimer derived from a different IgG4 molecule. Therefore, whereas the original IgG4 antibody was bivalent and monospecific for its antigen, the process of HL exchange results in a hybrid IgG4 that is monovalent for the original antigen and bispecific. Since most naturally occurring IgG4 has been reported to be bispecific [44], it has been suggested that even those IgG4 molecules that do have disulfide bonds between the heavy chains may be susceptible to HL exchange due to conversion of inter-heavy-chain bonds to intra-heavy-chain bonds by *in vivo* isomerase enzymes. This whole phenomenon can be avoided for IgG4s by introducing a single Ser to Pro amino acid substitution in the hinge (giving it the same core hinge sequence as IgG1) that enables efficient and stable disulfide bonding between heavy chains [45].

Amino Acid Sequence Variants

As suggested above, the improved understanding of the downstream events associated with binding to the different FcγRs has led to efforts to enhance antibody-effector function by identifying antibody variants that show preferential binding to activating receptors over the inhibiting receptor. By systematically changing each solvent-exposed amino acid in the Fc domain of human IgG1 and studying the effects on binding to different FcγRs, Shields et al. [46] identified various mutations that either enhanced affinity for an activating FcγR, or reduced affinity for the inhibiting FcγR, or both. Importantly, enhanced FcγR binding was shown to translate into greater activity in *in vitro* ADCC assays. Although the increases or decreases in affinity for the different FcγRs were modest in these earliest surveys of mutant IgGs, such data showed that numerous mutations in antibodies did not affect all FcγRs in the same way, and therefore provided optimism that more extensive searches for antibody variants could yield much more potent sequences that confer whichever FcγR binding profile was sought for a particular therapeutic antibody.

Fc Glycan Optimization

A different approach to enhancing antibody-effector functions entails optimizing the structure of the asparagine-linked glycan attached in the IgG Fc domain. It has been known for some time that antibodies that have been enzymatically deglycosylated, or genetically mutated so that they do not get glycosylated at that site, have a dramatically reduced affinity for FcγRs. The IgG Fc glycan structure, enveloped to a considerable extent between the two Fc-domain protein backbones, apparently plays a critical role in defining the conformation of the FcγR-binding site. More recently it has been learned that the presence of particular glycan structures (glycoforms) can dramatically increase the affinity of the antibody for particular FcγRs. For example, compared with IgG antibodies with Fc glycans that have maximal levels of the sugar fucose, IgG antibodies with Fc glycans that lack fucose have been reported to have 50-fold greater affinity for FcγR CD16 [47]. The relevance of this increased affinity has been demonstrated in *in vitro* ADCC assays in which a fucosylated antibody has been shown to be 100-fold more effective than a fully fucosylated version of the same antibody at triggering lysis of antigen-expressing target cells by CD16-express-ing immune-effector cells [47–49]. Another glycan manipulation that has been shown to enhance ADCC activity of antibodies at least 100-fold involves coexpression of antibodies with the enzyme β(1,4)-*N*-acetylglucosaminyltransferase III [50]. This enzyme attaches a bisecting *N*-acetylglucosamine sugar residue to the Fc glycan, which itself has a beneficial effect on ADCC activity, but the enzymatic activity also results in reduced levels of fucose being attached.

More recently, lower levels of the sugar sialic acid in the Fc glycan have been reported to be associated with proinflammatory properties and greater binding to at least some FcγRs, including CD16A on NK cells [51, 52]. The greater binding to CD16A on NK cells correlated with enhanced ADCC activity *in vitro*. Interestingly, for at least some antibodies, reduced levels of sialic acid were also associated with tighter binding to cell-surface antigen, suggesting that enhanced ADCC activity of lesser sialylated antibodies could be due to a combination of enhanced binding to FcγR on the immune-effector cells and enhanced binding to antigen on the target cells [52]. Interestingly, the various FcγRs are not all sensitive to the same structural variations, e.g., whereas CD16 binding is highly sensitive to fucose content, CD64 binding does not appear to be impacted by fucose content. Fc glycan engineering provides another means to optimize the immune-effector functions of antibodies, and several companies are pursuing such a strategy by developing host production cells engineered to express specific glycoforms. It remains to be seen to what extent having optimized Fc glycan structures added to an antibody already optimized for amino acid sequence will enhance ADCC potency even further. It also remains to be seen whether optimization of antibodies based on *in vitro* activity will translate into improved clinical efficacy while minimizing undesired effects.

THE FcγR-DEPENDENT AVIDITY EFFECT

Clearly, when it comes to FcγR binding, most attention tends to be focused on defined immune-effector functions, such as ADCC. But FcγR binding can also confer a potent avidity effect on the antibody for its antigen, at least in those cases where antigen is on the surface of a cell or is otherwise immobilized, perhaps in a soluble, polyvalent complex. Those antibody molecules bound to antigen on the surface of one cell and simultaneously bound to FcγR on the surface of a neighboring cell are likely to have a much slower rate of dissociation from antigen than antibody molecules that are not bound to FcγR. This is because FcγR binding serves to keep the antibody molecules in the immediate vicinity even after dissociation from antigen, making it more likely that they will then reassociate with antigen. In addition to enhancing the effective affinity for antigen, depending on the antigen target, such simultaneous FcγR binding may have biological implications, as has been described for anti-CD3 antibodies that bind T cells [53, 54].

ENHANCED COMPLEMENT ACTIVITY

Another well-known immune-effector function of IgG antibodies is CDC. The cascade of enzymatic events in the classical pathway of complement activation is triggered by the binding of C1q complement protein to a cluster of IgG1 or IgG3 (or IgM) Fc domains. In the case of therapeutic antibodies bound to tumor cells, the pathway would ideally culminate in the lysis of the tumor cell by the newly formed membrane-attack complex of the complement. However, because mammalian cells, including tumor cells, express significant amounts of membrane complement regulatory proteins (mCRP) — e.g., CD46, CD55, and CD59 — that can inhibit the complement cascade at specific stages, the contribution of complement-mediated lysis to antibody-triggered cytotoxicity of tumors has been somewhat questionable. Efforts are ongoing to block the complement inhibition effect of these mCRPs by cotreatment with an anti-mCRP blocking antibody in addition to the antitumor-specific antibody [55]. Fortunately, recent data suggest that even if complement-mediated tumor cell lysis in response to antibody therapy is minimal, other beneficial effects of progressing at least part way through the complement cascade may be realized through mobilization of cellular inflammatory responses induced by intermediate-stage complement products [56]. Large numbers of complement protein iC3b have been shown to be deposited on tumor targets following rituximab (IgG1) binding [57], and iC3b molecules on such targets may then bind CD11b/CD18 on macrophages and NK cells to activate CDCC, a killing mechanism distinct from CDC. Consequently, antibody variants that show increased affinity for C1q, at least enough to initiate the complement cascade regardless of whether the complement membrane-attack complex gets formed in sufficient numbers, are becoming of greater interest.

The ongoing focus to enhance immune-effector functions of antibodies through engineering their amino acid sequence or their Fc glycan structure holds much promise. Yet it seems likely that other novel structures will eventually be engineered that offer even more advantages, e.g., by engaging immune-effector cells such as neutrophils that are not recruited by current antibody constructs.

IMMUNOCONJUGATES AS CANCER THERAPEUTICS

Immunoconjugates are a distinct class of therapeutics in oncology. They are bifunctional molecules that combine the specificity of monoclonal antibodies to tumor antigens with the extraordinary potency of cytotoxic agents. Generally, an immunoconjugate consists of three moieties: a specific tumor-targeting antibody or a functional fragment of antibodies such as a nanobody [58]; a cytotoxic agent, which can be a small molecular drug, a protein toxin, or a radioisotope molecule; and a linker, which covalently or noncovalently links the targeting agent and cytotoxic agent together. Immunoconjugates can be classified into three subgroups: (a) antibody–drug conjugates, if the cytotoxin is a small-molecule drug, (b) immunotoxins, if a protein toxin is used as the cytotoxic agent, and (c) radioimmunoconjugates, if the targeting molecule is labeled with a radioisotope. Under certain circumstances, drug–antibody immunoconjugates are also called tumor-activated prodrugs (TAP) [59]. There are a number of comprehensive reviews of immunoconjugates [60–63]. In this section, discussions will be focused on the concept of antibody–drug conjugates and their current progress as cancer therapeutics.

TARGETING MOLECULE

The selection of the "ideal" targeting molecule is crucial for delivering a selective cytotoxic agent to cancer cells. Complete sequencing of the human genome and application of proteomic tools in discovery of new cancer biomarkers provide valuable approaches to identify new targets for cancer therapy. The basic concept for identification of tumor-associated antigens and selection of potential therapeutic targets has been discussed in detail [64–67]. A tumor antigen targeted by immunoconjugates should be a cell-surface protein with selective expression in tumor tissues (tumor-specific antigen) or at least with high expression levels in tumors relative to normal tissues (selective tumor antigen). The tumor antigen chosen as target would also be one that internalizes after being bound by antibody. Internalization of the antigen–immunoconjugate complex would be followed by intracellular cleavage of the linker, leading to release of active, cytotoxic drug.

A large number of tumor-associated antigens have been selected as targets for immunoconjugates. These include receptor tyrosine kinases such as EGFR and HER2 [68], mucins such as CanAg [69], integrin $\alpha v \beta 3$ [70], and selectins such as E-selectin [71]. In most cases, because the tumor antigen is likely to be expressed by normal tissues, it is important to balance the relative selectivity of the targeting molecule with the potency of the agent delivered.

CYTOTOXINS

Many cytotoxic chemotherapeutic agents — bacterial and plant toxins or their derivatives — have been conjugated to targeting antibodies. The selection of potent cytotoxic agents is another key factor in successfully developing potent antibody–drug conjugates. To choose a cytotoxic drug for immunoconjugation, several factors must be kept in mind. First, with current technologies, only three to ten drug molecules can be linked to an antibody, and thus the ratio of drug to antibody is

TABLE 5.2
Typical Cytotoxic Agents Used in Immunoconjugates

Name	Target	Example	Reference
Auristatin	Microtubule	anti-CD30–Auristatin E	[88]
Calicheamicin	DNA	anti-CD33–Calicheamicin	[115]
Doxorubicin	DNA/telomerase	anti-Lewis Y–Doxorubicin	[121]
DM1	Microtubule	anti-CanAg–DM1	[69]
Pseudomonas exotoxin A	Elongation factor 2	anti-CD22–PE38	[122]
Iodine-131 (^{131}I)	DNA	^{131}I–anti-CD20	[123]
Yttrium-90 (^{90}Y)	DNA	^{90}Y–anti-CD20	[124]

low. Second, tumor-antigen densities on the cell surface are usually between 10^5 and 10^7 molecules per cell. Therefore, the number of binding sites for a particular antibody–drug conjugate may be limited. Third, the efficiency of processes such as endocytosis of antigen–immunoconjugate complexes and drug release from the lysosome or other intracellular compartments is usually not 100%. Thus, it has been hypothesized that only cytotoxins with potencies (as defined by *in vitro* assays) in the picomolar to nanomolar range are useful in generating immunoconjugates [72, 73]. Some potent cytotoxic agents used in immunoconjugates are listed in Table 5.2, and they include small-molecule drugs, protein toxins, and radioisotopes.

LINKER

The nature of the linker between the cytotoxic agent and the targeting antibody (or functional fragments of antibodies) dictates the degree of successful delivery and release of cytotoxic agents. Ideal linkers should meet two essential criteria: they must be stable in systemic circulation, but they must be specifically cleaved when internalized into cells. Immunoconjugates are macromolecular drugs. Like any other macromolecule, the immunoconjugate will be up taken by cells via an endocytic pathway such as pinocytosis [74] or clathrin-mediated pathways [75]. There exist alternative routes for the uptake of macromolecules, such as caveolae-mediated processes [76], but their roles are still unclear and might be minor. Once taken up by cells, immunoconjugates are first in the endosomal compartment. Then the endocytosed immunoconjugates will be either recirculated back to the cell surface or further transferred into the acidic (pH 4.5–5.0) lysosomal compartment, which contains enzymes that are able to degrade immunoconjugates and release drugs such as hydrolases, peptidases, and thioredoxin enzymes. A variety of linkers have been developed and used in conjugation of antibodies with cytotoxic agents, and several are described here.

Acid-Labile Linkages

There is a pH gradient from the extracellular environment to intracellular compartments. The pH is 7.2–7.4 outside of cells, while the pH value is 6–6.8 in endosomes and 4.5–5.5 in lysosomes. It has also been reported that the tumor tissues are 0.5–1.0 pH units more acidic than normal tissues. Acid-labile linkers have been developed based on this information. For example, the antitumor drug doxorubicin was coupled to the low-molecular-weight protein lysozyme via the acid-sensitive *cis*-aconityl linker [77]. Results have demonstrated that the release of cytotoxic doxorubicin in the bladder can be achieved by acidification of the urine. Another type of acid-sensitive linker is the hydrazone linker, which has been broadly used in a number of drug conjugates, such as doxorubicin, 5-fluorouridine, and vinblastin. Mylotarg, an anti-CD33-calicheamicin conjugate targeting acute myeloid leukemia (AML), is the first antibody–drug conjugate approved by the FDA, the linker of which contains both a cleavable acylhydrazone bond and a disulfide bond [78].

Sulfhydryl Linkages

Many bacterial and plant toxins are composed of a toxic enzymatic subunit A that is covalently linked by a disulfide bond to a binding subunit B, such as pseudomonas exotoxin A, cholera toxin, or the plant toxin ricin. A key event in the intracellular activation of these A-B toxins is the reduction of the disulfide bond between subunit A and subunit B, followed by release of the cytotoxic subunit A [79]. This evidence demonstrates the importance of the disulfide bond in the activation of A-B toxins and also suggests that disulfide linkage is a possible way of releasing drugs from antibodies in intracellular compartments. The disulfide bond is intended to be cleaved once inside the target cell, but it has also been shown to be unstable in the circulation. *In vivo* instability of these linkages and the resulting release of active free toxin likely lead to general toxicity and reduced tumor-specific cytotoxicity. Toxins and linkers with sterically hindered, stabler disulfide bonds have been developed to address this issue [80].

The manner in which a cytotoxic drug is released inside a cell from a conjugate with a disulfide bond linker remains elusive. Recently, Erickson and colleagues [81] examined the metabolic fate in cells of huC242-SPDB-DM4, which has a disulfide linker, and huC242-SMCC-DM1, which has a thioether linker, using cell-cycle analysis combined with lysosomal inhibitors. They demonstrated that lysosomal processing is required for the activity of antibody–maytansinoid conjugates, irrespective of the linker. Regarding cleavage of the disulfide bond, it has been proposed that cysteine is the physiological reducing agent within the endosomal compartment. However, the mechanism of reduction of a disulfide bond within cells remains unclear. A recent review by Saito et al. [82] discussed in detail where and how the disulfide bond in immunoconjugates is reduced upon entering cells. In eukaryotic cells, the ubiquitous thioredoxin system (thioredoxin + thioredoxin reductase) [83] and the glutaredoxin system (glutaredoxin + glutaredoxin reductase) [84] catalyze fast and reversible thiodisulfide exchanges between cysteines in their active site and cysteines of their disulfide substrates. The newly discovered gamma-interferon-inducible lysosomal thioreductase (GILT) is the first reducing enzyme identified mainly in the endocytic pathway [85, 86]. Unlike other thioreductases, GILT has unique characteristics. The optimal pH for GILT activity is 4.0–5.5, in contrast to neutral pH for other thioreductases [87]. The discovery of GILT may provide, at least in part, an explanation of how a disulfide bond is broken up in a very acidic environment.

Several immunoconjugates in which the antibody and drug are linked by a disulfide linkage have been developed. As mentioned above, the linker for Mylotarg (anti-CD33-calicheamicin) contains a disulfide bond as well as an acid-labile hydrazone bond [78]. Other antibody–drug conjugates at late development stages include huC242-DM4 (anti-CanAg-DM4) and huMy9-6-DM4 (AVE9633, anti-CD33-DM4) [63].

Enzyme-Degradable Linkages

Enzyme-degradable linkers have also been designed. These linkers often have a peptide sequence that is sensitive to cleavage by lysosomal enzymes [88, 89] or tumor-associated enzymes [90]. For example, doxorubicin has been conjugated to anti-Lewis Y monoclonal antibody through linkers consisting of cleavable dipeptides Phe-Lys or Val-Cit. Both conjugates demonstrated rapid and near-quantitative doxorubicin release when incubated with either the cysteine protease cathepsin B or in a rat liver lysosomal preparation [89]. These immunoconjugates also demonstrated significant antitumor activity against a lung carcinoma expressing Lewis Y antigen. An anti-CD30 antibody, cAC-10, has been linked with monomethyl auristatin E, a synthetic analog of the natural product dolastatin 10, by a linker containing Val-Cit peptide. This immunoconjugate has been demonstrated to be highly potent and selective against CD30+ tumor cell lines. In SCID mouse xenograft models of anaplastic large-cell lymphoma or Hodgkin's disease, cAC-10–auristatin E conjugate was efficacious at doses as low as 1 mg/kg [88]. Considering its maximal tolerated dose is more than 30 mg/kg, it is apparent that cAC-10–auristatin E conjugate possesses a wide therapeutic window.

Efforts have been made to increase drug loading onto antibodies. For example, branched linkers have been developed allowing the loading of multiple drug molecules on a single targeting antibody. This technology leads to enhanced conjugate potency [91]. To date, three immunoconjugates have been approved by the FDA and are marketed, including Mylotarg, Zevalin, and Bexxar. All of them are used to treat hematological cancers. This is a landmark in immunoconjugate development.

ENHANCING DRUG DELIVERY THROUGH LIGAND-TARGETED LIPOSOMES

Many cancer therapeutics are potent cytotoxins, but systemic delivery of these drugs results in cytotoxic activity against both the tumor cells and healthy cells throughout the body. Exposure of healthy cells to cytotoxins causes undesirable side effects that limit drug dose or dosing frequency, and this ultimately constrains drug efficacy and tumor control. Strategies that increase the therapeutic index of such drugs and reduce their toxicity to the patient are highly desirable. Ligand-targeted liposomes (LTL) are one way in which the biodistribution and uptake of a cancer drug can be altered favorably to achieve these goals. LTLs also represent another strategy by which the targeting power of antibodies can help create more-effective anticancer therapeutics.

Tumors differ in many ways from normal tissues, but one key difference that can be exploited by liposome technologies is that tumor vasculature is defective and leaky. Normal blood vessels consist of endothelial cells with tight junctions that do not permit liposomes to extravasate to neighboring tissue. However, the vessels in tumors are permeable, with pores that range from 100 to 800 nm in diameter. This raised the possibility that small liposomes, on the order of 60 to 150 nm, could traverse the tumor vasculature and deliver toxic payloads directly to the tumor. In addition, tumors lack lymphatic drainage, so liposomes are not readily cleared from the tumor and can continue to accumulate.

Liposomes are composed of phospholipid bilayers that enclose an aqueous inner compartment. Usually the inner compartment is formulated to contain a hydrophilic payload, but hydrophobic drugs can be associated with the lipid bilayer. Initial experiments with "naked" liposomes injected intravenously (i.v.) showed that liposomes were cleared within minutes from the bloodstream [92, 93]. It was found that serum proteins adsorbed to the liposome surface, which caused leakage and loss of integrity of the liposome [94–96]. In addition, adhesion of serum proteins led to recognition and uptake by the mononuclear phagocyte system (MPS), primarily macrophages in the liver and spleen, which led to rapid liposome clearance. Finally, antibodies may recognize directly the lipid bilayer and facilitate the removal of liposomes from the bloodstream [97, 98].

To address the limitations of naked liposomes, many attempts were made to shield the liposome from the MPS. It was found that the half-life of liposomes could be greatly increased by coating the liposome surface with a hydrophilic carbohydrate or polymer, such as polyethylene glycol (PEG) [99, 100]. The PEG coating is thought to sterically stabilize the liposomal membrane and resist interaction with serum proteins. PEG-coated liposomes evade recognition by the MPS, and thus their half-life is extended from minutes to many hours, up to 20 hours in mice [101] and 45 hours in humans [102]. These PEG-coated liposomes, known as Stealth® liposomes, have shown greater efficacy than free drug in tumor models. Approved Stealth liposomal drugs include Doxil®/Caelyx®, Myocet®, and Daunosome®, and there are many other Stealth liposome drug candidates in clinical trials [103].

Doxil is an interesting example of the positive impact of formulating a cytotoxic (doxorubicin) in a Stealth liposome. Doxorubicin's half-life in vivo is on the order of minutes, while that of Doxil is many hours. More importantly, up to 10% of an injected dose of Doxil accumulates in patients' tumors, which is about tenfold higher than the accumulation of free drug [104]. The side-effect profiles of each drug are also quite different. Patients receiving doxorubicin experience myelosuppression, alopecia, and nausea, and there is significant risk of cardiotoxicity with cumulative dosing. The latter side effect ultimately limits administration of the drug, though doxorubicin continues to have antitumor activity. In contrast, Doxil's primary dose-limiting side effect is skin swelling and redness (palmar/plantar erythrodysesthesia [PPE]), with stomatitis and nausea also observed, but no cardiotoxicity. The dermatologic side effect occurs because liposomes traverse the lymphatics and accumulate in the skin, in addition to extravasation in the tumor vasculature. The key message is that the efficacy of doxorubicin and its side-effect profile are improved through the Stealth formulation.

LTLs further refine Stealth liposomes by insertion of a tumor-targeting ligand into the lipid bilayer. Stealth liposomes allow drug accumulation and release near tumor cells, but a targeting moiety on the liposome could facilitate internalization and drug release within tumor cells, which could lead to greater efficacy. The most popular ligands include antibodies and antibody fragments (Stealth immunoliposomes), though other ligands are used as well. One concern about LTLs is the potential for development of an immune response to the LTL. Early experiments with whole IgG inserted into Stealth liposomes demonstrated rapid clearance from the bloodstream, which was likely due to recognition of the Fc portion of the antibody by the MPS [105]. When single-chain Fv (scFv) or Fab′ fragments that lack the Fc were used instead as targeting moieties, the half-life of the Stealth immunoliposome was restored to that of Stealth liposomes. Thus it is possible to design appropriate ligands that allow retention of the desirable half-life shown by Stealth liposomes.

A key question to address is whether the presence of a targeting ligand impacts the biodistribution of the liposome, particularly because most, if not all, ligands will recognize receptors abundantly present on tumor tissue and at lower levels on normal tissue. Studies have shown that LTLs and Stealth liposomes accumulate to similar levels in tumors [106, 107], indicating that the biodistribution of the drug is determined by the liposome carrier, with minimal influence of the targeting agent. Once the LTL reaches the tumor, however, internalization of the drug can be demonstrated, in contrast to Stealth liposomes that remain on the tumor periphery [106, 107]. Thus, this novel drug class exhibits both passive targeting based on the liposome carrier and active targeting based on the targeting ligand. An additional advantage is that the toxicity of LTLs should be predictable based on the biodistribution of Stealth liposomes.

The way the targeting ligand is inserted into the liposome has an impact on the efficacy of the molecule. Targeting ligands can be attached in two ways to the liposome, either inserted directly into the liposome bilayer, or attached to the distal end of the PEG chain (pendant type). The latter approach makes the targeting ligand more available for interaction with its receptor, and this appears to result in greater binding to target *in vivo* [108]. Other characteristics of the targeting ligand also impact efficacy. For example, higher valence (30–50 targeting molecules per liposome) appears to enhance binding to tumor *in vivo* [108]. However, higher avidity may not be an advantage, as high-avidity LTL may bind preferentially to the first tumor cells encountered at the periphery of the tumor ("binding site barrier" hypothesis [109]). Lower-avidity targeting molecules may enable better penetration of the tumor interior. Finally, studies suggest that the tumor cell itself should express at least 10^4–10^5 copies of the receptor to aid binding and internalization of the LTL [110, 111].

Most importantly, LTLs have shown increased efficacy in preclinical tumor models as compared with nontargeted Stealth liposomes. For example, LTLs designed with antibody fragments specific for CD19 [111], Her2 [107, 110], and B1 integrins [112], among others, all show significantly enhanced antitumor activity compared with nontargeted liposomes. The increased efficacy observed with LTLs in multiple model systems strongly suggests that this advance in liposome technology may have clinical benefit, and it is expected that such novel drugs will soon move into clinical trials.

CONCLUSIONS

Therapeutic antibodies are currently providing clinical benefits to many patients suffering with cancer. Many other antibodies are in late-stage clinical development, providing optimism that more patients will benefit from antibody therapy in the future. Antibodies marketed and in development have been selected on the basis of their tumor specificity or their mechanism of action, and many have been termed "targeted therapies" because they are selective and have marginal effects on non-cancerous cells. The field of informatics hopes to provide us with more cancer-specific targets and biomarkers to select patients that will respond to these therapies. In addition, informatics can also help to advance antibody technologies, such as Fc engineering and antibody/payload conjugation, to provide even more effective anti-body-based drugs that will help to convert cancer into a manageable and chronic — rather than fatal — disease.

REFERENCES

1. Kohler, G., Milstein, C. Continuous cultures of fused cells secreting antibody of predefined specificity. *Nature* 1975; 256 (5517): 495–7.
2. Ezzell, C. Magic bullets fly again. *Sci. Am.* 2001; 285 (4): 34–41.
3. Carter, P. Improving the efficacy of antibody-based cancer therapies. *Nat. Rev. Cancer* 2001; 1 (2): 118–29.
4. Zwick, E., Bange, J., Ullrich, A. Receptor tyrosine kinases as targets for anticancer drugs. *Trends Mol. Med.* 2002; 8 (1): 17–23.
5. Klement, G., Huang, P., Mayer, B., et al. Differences in therapeutic indexes of combination metronomic chemotherapy and an anti-VEGFR-2 antibody in multidrug-resistant human breast cancer xenografts. *Clin. Cancer Res.* 2002; 8 (1): 221–32.
6. Hurwitz, H., Fehrenbacher, L., Novotny, W., et al. Bevacizumab plus irinotecan, fluorouracil, and leucovorin for metastatic colorectal cancer. *N. Engl. J. Med.* 2004; 350 (23): 2335–42.
7. Saltz, L.B., Meropol, N.J., Loehrer, P.J., Sr., Needle, M.N., Kopit, J., Mayer, R.J. Phase II trial of cetuximab in patients with refractory colorectal cancer that expresses the epidermal growth factor receptor. *J. Clin. Oncol.* 2004; 22 (7): 1201–8.
8. Folkman, J., Browder, T., Palmblad, J. Angiogenesis research: guidelines for translation to clinical application. *Thromb. Haemost.* 2001; 86 (1): 23–33.
9. Posey, J.A., Khazaeli, M.B., DelGrosso, A., et al. A pilot trial of Vitaxin, a humanized anti-vitronectin receptor (anti alpha v beta 3) antibody in patients with metastatic cancer. *Cancer Biother. Radiopharm.* 2001; 16 (2): 125–32.
10. Jayson, G.C., Mullamitha, S., Ton, C., et al. Phase I study of CNTO 95, a fully human monoclonal antibody (mAb) to v integrins, in patients with solid tumors. In *Annual Meeting Proceedings of the American Society of Clinical Oncology* 2004; 23: 224.
11. Bissell, M.J., Radisky, D. Putting tumours in context. *Nat. Rev. Cancer* 2001; 1 (1): 46–54.
12. Yan, L., Song, X.-Y., Nakada, M. Interplay between inflammation and tumor angiogenesis. In: Morgan, D., Forssman, U.J., Nakada, M., eds. *Cancer and Inflammation.* Basel: Birkhauser Publishing; 2004: 99–121.

13. Maisey, N.R., Hall, K., Lee, C., et al. Infliximab: a phase II trial of the tumour necrosis factor (TNF) monoclonal antibody in patients with advanced renal cell cancer (RCC). In *Annual Meeting Proceedings of the American Society of Clinical Oncology* 2004; 23: 384.

14. Anderson, G., Nakada, M., DeWitte, M. Tumor necrosis factor-a in the pathogenesis and treatment of cancer. *Curr. Opinion Pharmacol.* 2004; 4: 314–20.

15. Kurzrock, R. The role of cytokines in cancer-related fatigue. *Cancer* 2001; 92 (6 Suppl.): 1684–8.

16. Wichers, M., Maes, M. The psychoneuroimmuno-pathophysiology of cytokine-induced depression in humans. *Int. J. Neuropsychopharmacol.* 2002; 5 (4): 375–88.

17. Ramesh, G., Reeves, W.B. TNF-alpha mediates chemokine and cytokine expression and renal injury in cisplatin nephrotoxicity. *J. Clin. Invest.* 2002; 110 (6): 835–42.

18. Tobinick, E.L. Targeted etanercept for treatment-refractory pain due to bone metastasis: two case reports. *Clin. Ther.* 2003; 25 (8): 2279–88.

19. Korngold, R., Marini, J.C., de Baca, M.E., Murphy, G.F., Giles-Komar, J. Role of tumor necrosis factor-alpha in graft-versus-host disease and graft-versus-leukemia responses. *Biol. Blood Marrow Transplant* 2003; 9 (5): 292–303.

20. Tisdale, M.J., Cachexia in cancer patients. *Nat. Rev. Cancer* 2002; 2 (11): 862–71.

21. Guttridge, D.C., Mayo, M.W., Madrid, L.V., Wang, C.Y., Baldwin, A.S., Jr. NF-kappa B-induced loss of MyoD messenger RNA: possible role in muscle decay and cachexia. *Science* 2000; 289 (5488): 2363–6.

22. Acharyya, S., Ladner, K.J., Nelsen, L.L., et al. Cancer cachexia is regulated by selective targeting of skeletal muscle gene products. *J. Clin. Invest.* 2004; 114 (3): 370–8.

23. Argiles, J.M., Busquets, S., Lopez-Soriano, F.J. Cytokines in the pathogenesis of cancer cachexia. *Curr. Opinion Clin. Nutr. Metab. Care* 2003; 6 (4): 401–6.

24. Azuma, Y., Kaji, K., Katogi, R., Takeshita, S., Kudo, A. Tumor necrosis factor-alpha induces differentiation of and bone resorption by osteoclasts. *J. Biol. Chem.* 2000; 275 (7): 4858–64.

25. Schafers, M., Lee, D.H., Brors, D., Yaksh, T.L., Sorkin, L.S. Increased sensitivity of injured and adjacent uninjured rat primary sensory neurons to exogenous tumor necrosis factor-alpha after spinal nerve ligation. *J. Neurosci.* 2003; 23 (7): 3028–38.

26. Delanian, S., Porcher, R., Balla-Mekias, S., Lefaix, J.L. Randomized, placebo-controlled trial of combined pentoxifylline and tocopherol for regression of superficial radiation-induced fibrosis. *J. Clin. Oncol.* 2003; 21 (13): 2545–50.

27. Rube, C.E., van Valen, F., Wilfert, F., et al. Ewing's sarcoma and peripheral primitive neuroectodermal tumor cells produce large quantities of bioactive tumor necrosis factor-alpha (TNF-alpha) after radiation exposure. *Int. J. Radiat. Oncol. Biol. Phys.* 2003; 56 (5): 1414–25.

28. Best, C.J., Emmert-Buck, M.R. Molecular profiling of tissue samples using laser capture microdissection. *Expert Rev. Mol. Diagn.* 2001; 1 (1): 53–60.

29. Liotta, L.A., Kohn, E.C., Petricoin, E.F. Clinical proteomics: personalized molecular medicine. *JAMA* 2001; 286 (18): 2211–4.

30. Liu, B., Huang, L., Sihlbom, C., Burlingame, A., Marks, J.D. Towards proteome-wide production of monoclonal antibody by phage display. *J. Mol. Biol.* 2002; 315 (5): 1063–73.

31. Agus, D.B., Akita, R.W., Fox, W.D., et al. Targeting ligand-activated ErbB2 signaling inhibits breast and prostate tumor growth. *Cancer Cell* 2002; 2 (2): 127–37.

32. Albanell, J., Codony, J., Rovira, A., Mellado, B., Gascon, P. Mechanism of action of anti-HER2 monoclonal antibodies: scientific update on trastuzumab and 2C4. *Adv. Exp. Med. Biol.* 2003; 532: 253–68.

33. Ravetch, J.V., Bolland, S. IgG Fc receptors. *Annu. Rev. Immunol.* 2001; 19: 275–90.

34. Dijstelbloem, H.M., van de Winkel, J.G., Kallenberg, C.G. Inflammation in autoimmunity: receptors for IgG revisited. *Trends Immunol.* 2001; 22 (9): 510–6.

35. Harrison, P.T., Davis, W., Norman, J.C., Hockaday, A.R., Allen, J.M. Binding of monomeric immunoglobulin G triggers Fc gamma RI-mediated endocytosis. *J. Biol. Chem.* 1994; 269 (39): 24396–402.

36. Guyre, C.A., Keler, T., Swink, S.L., Vitale, L.A., Graziano, R.F., Fanger, M.W. Receptor modulation by Fc gamma RI-specific fusion proteins is dependent on receptor number and modified by IgG. *J. Immunol.* 2001; 167 (11): 6303–11.

37. Clynes, R.A., Towers, T.L., Presta, L.G., Ravetch, J.V. Inhibitory Fc receptors modulate in vivo cytoxicity against tumor targets. *Nat. Med.* 2000; 6 (4): 443–6.

38. Cartron, G., Dacheux, L., Salles, G., et al. Therapeutic activity of humanized anti-CD20 monoclonal antibody and polymorphism in IgG Fc receptor Fcgamma RIIIa gene. *Blood* 2002; 99 (3): 754–8.

39. Weng, W.K., Levy, R. Two immunoglobulin G fragment C receptor polymorphisms independently predict response to rituximab in patients with follicular lymphoma. *J. Clin. Oncol.* 2003; 21 (21): 3940–7.

40. Dall'Ozzo, S., Tartas, S., Paintaud, G., et al. Rituximab-dependent cytotoxicity by natural killer cells: influence of FCGR3A polymorphism on the concentration-effect relationship. *Cancer Res.* 2004; 64 (13): 4664–9.

41. Isaacs, J.D., Wing, M.G., Greenwood, J.D., Hazleman, B.L., Hale, G., Waldmann, H. A therapeutic human IgG4 monoclonal antibody that depletes target cells in humans. *Clin. Exp. Immunol.* 1996; 106 (3): 427–33.

42. Bolt, S., Routledge, E., Lloyd, I., et al. The generation of a humanized, non-mitogenic CD3 monoclonal antibody which retains in vitro immunosuppressive properties. *Eur. J. Immunol.* 1993; 23 (2): 403–11.

43. Aalberse, R.C., Schuurman, J. IgG4 breaking the rules. *Immunology* 2002; 105 (1): 9–19.

44. Schuurman, J., Van Ree, R., Perdok, G.J., Van Doorn, H.R., Tan, K.Y., Aalberse, R.C. Normal human immunoglobulin G4 is bispecific: it has two different antigen-combining sites. *Immunology* 1999; 97 (4): 693–8.

45. Angal, S., King, D.J., Bodmer, M.W., et al. A single amino acid substitution abolishes the heterogeneity of chimeric mouse/human (IgG4) antibody. *Mol. Immunol.* 1993; 30 (1): 105–8.

46. Shields, R.L., Namenuk, A.K., Hong, K., et al. High resolution mapping of the binding site on human IgG1 for Fc gamma RI, Fc gamma RII, Fc gamma RIII, and FcRn and design of IgG1 variants with improved binding to the Fc gamma R. *J. Biol. Chem.* 2001; 276 (9): 6591–604.

47. Shields, R.L., Lai, J., Keck, R., et al. Lack of fucose on human IgG1 N-linked oligosaccharide improves binding to human Fc gamma RIII and antibody-dependent cellular toxicity. *J. Biol. Chem.* 2002; 277 (30): 26733–40.

48. Shinkawa, T., Nakamura, K., Yamane, N., et al. The absence of fucose but not the presence of galactose or bisecting N-acetylglucosamine of human IgG1 complex-type oligosaccharides shows the critical role of enhancing antibody-dependent cellular cytotoxicity. *J. Biol. Chem.* 2003; 278 (5): 3466–73.

49. Yamane-Ohnuki, N., Kinoshita, S., Inoue-Urakubo, M., et al. Establishment of FUT8 knockout Chinese hamster ovary cells: an ideal host cell line for producing completely defucosylated antibodies with enhanced antibody-dependent cellular cytotoxicity. *Biotechnol. Bioeng.* 2004; 87 (5): 614–22.

50. Umana, P., Jean-Mairet, J., Moudry, R., Amstutz, H., Bailey, J.E. Engineered glycoforms of an antineuroblastoma IgG1 with optimized antibody-dependent cellular cytotoxic activity. *Nat. Biotechnol.* 1999; 17 (2): 176–80.

51. Kaneko, Y., Nimmerjahn, F., Ravetch, J.V. Anti-inflammatory activity of immunoglobulin G resulting from Fc sialylation. *Science* 2006; 313 (5787): 670–3.

52. Scallon, B.J., Tam, S.H., McCarthy, S.G., Cai, A.N., Raju, T.S. Higher levels of sialylated Fc glycans in immunoglobulin G molecules can adversely impact functionality. *Mol. Immunol.*, 2007; 44: 1524–1534.

53. Herold, K.C., Burton, J.B., Francois, F., Poumian-Ruiz, E., Glandt, M., Bluestone, J.A. Activation of human T cells by FcR nonbinding anti-CD3 mAb, hOKT3gamma1 (Ala-Ala). *J. Clin. Invest.* 2003; 111 (3): 409–18.

54. Carpenter, P.A., Pavlovic, S., Tso, J.Y., et al. Non-Fc receptor-binding humanized anti-CD3 antibodies induce apoptosis of activated human T cells. *J. Immunol.* 2000; 165 (11): 6205–13.

55. Fishelson, Z., Donin, N., Zell, S., Schultz, S., Kirschfink, M. Obstacles to cancer immunotherapy: expression of membrane complement regulatory proteins (mCRPs) in tumors. *Mol. Immunol.* 2003; 40 (2–4): 109–23.

56. Bergman, I., Basse, P.H., Barmada, M.A., Griffin, J.A., Cheung, N.K. Comparison of in vitro antibody-targeted cytotoxicity using mouse, rat and human effectors. *Cancer Immunol. Immunother.* 2000; 49 (4–5): 259–66.

57. Kennedy, A.D., Solga, M.D., Schuman, T.A., et al. An anti-C3b(i) mAb enhances complement activation, C3b(i) deposition, and killing of CD20+ cells by rituximab. *Blood* 2003; 101 (3): 1071–9.

58. Cortez-Retamozo, V., Backmann, N., Senter, P.D., et al. Efficient cancer therapy with a nanobody-based conjugate. *Cancer Res.* 2004; 64 (8): 2853–7.

59. Blättler, W.A., Chari, R.V.J., Lambert, J.M. Immunoconjugates. In: Teicher, B.A., ed. *Cancer Therapeutics: Experimental and Clinical Agents.* Totowa, NJ: Humana Press; 1996: 371–94.

60. Garnett, M.C. Targeted drug conjugates: principles and progress. *Adv. Drug Deliv. Rev.* 2001; 53 (2): 171–216.

61. Payne, G. Progress in immunoconjugate cancer therapeutics. *Cancer Cell* 2003; 3 (3): 207–12.

62. Dyba, M., Tarasova, N.I., Michejda, C.J. Small molecule toxins targeting tumor receptors. *Curr. Pharm. Des.* 2004; 10 (19): 2311–34.

63. Lambert, J.M. Drug-conjugated monoclonal antibodies for the treatment of cancer. *Curr. Opinion Pharmacol.* 2005; 5 (5): 543–9.

64. Ilyin, S.E., Bernal, A., Horowitz, D., Derian, C.K., Xin, H. Functional informatics: convergence and integration of automation and bioinformatics. *Pharmacogenomics* 2004; 5 (6): 721–30.

65. Melle, C., Ernst, G., Schimmel, B., et al. A technical triade for proteomic identification and characterization of cancer biomarkers. *Cancer Res.* 2004; 64 (12): 4099–104.

66. Nicolette, C.A, Miller, G.A. The identification of clinically relevant markers and therapeutic targets. *Drug Discov. Today* 2003; 8 (1): 31–8.

67. Frank, R., Hargreaves, R. Clinical biomarkers in drug discovery and development. *Nat. Rev. Drug Discov.* 2003; 2 (7): 566–80.

68. Mandler, R., Kobayashi, H., Hinson, E.R., Brechbiel, M.W., Waldmann, T.A. Herceptin-geldanamycin immunoconjugates: pharmacokinetics, biodistribution, and enhanced antitumor activity. *Cancer Res.* 2004; 64 (4): 1460–7.

69. Liu, C., Tadayoni, B.M., Bourret, L.A., et al. Eradication of large colon tumor xenografts by targeted delivery of maytansinoids. *Proc. Natl. Acad. Sci. USA* 1996; 93 (16): 8618–23.

70. Hood, J.D., Bednarski, M., Frausto, R., et al. Tumor regression by targeted gene delivery to the neovasculature. *Science* 2002; 296 (5577): 2404–7.

71. Bhaskar, V., Law, D.A., Ibsen, E., et al. E-selectin up-regulation allows for targeted drug delivery in prostate cancer. *Cancer Res.* 2003; 63 (19): 6387–94.

72. Blättler, W.A., Chari, R.V.J. Drugs to enhance the therapeutic potency of anticancer antibodies: antibody-drug conjugates as tumor-activated prodrugs. In: Ojima, I., Vite, G.D., Altmann, K.-H., eds. *Anticancer Agents: Frontiers in Cancer Chemotherapy.* Washington, DC: American Chemical Society; 2001: 317–38.

73. Moody, T.W., Czerwinski, G., Tarasova, N.I., Michejda, C.J. VIP-ellipticine derivatives inhibit the growth of breast cancer cells. *Life Sci.* 2002; 71 (9): 1005–14.

74. Steinman, R.M., Silver, J.M., Cohn, Z.A. Pinocytosis in fibroblasts: quantitative studies in vitro. *J. Cell. Biol.* 1974; 63 (3): 949–69.

75. Goldstein, J.L., Anderson, R.G., Brown, M.S. Coated pits, coated vesicles, and receptor-mediated endocytosis. *Nature* 1979; 279 (5715): 679–85.

76. Parton, R.G., Simons, K. Digging into caveolae. *Science* 1995; 269 (5229): 1398–9.

77. Haas, M., Moolenaar, F., Elsinga, A., et al. Targeting of doxorubicin to the urinary bladder of the rat shows increased cytotoxicity in the bladder urine combined with an absence of renal toxicity. *J. Drug Target* 2002; 10 (1): 81–9.

78. Hamann, P.R., Hinman, L.M., Beyer, C.F., et al. An anti-CD33 antibody-calicheamicin conjugate for treatment of acute myeloid leukemia: choice of linker. *Bioconjug. Chem.* 2002; 13 (1): 40–6.

79. Falnes, P.O., Sandvig, K. Penetration of protein toxins into cells. *Curr. Opinion Cell. Biol.* 2000; 12 (4): 407–13.

80. Widdison, W.C., Wilhelm, S.D., Cavanagh, E.E., et al. Semisynthetic maytansine analogues for the targeted treatment of cancer. *J. Med. Chem.* 2006; 49 (14): 4392–408.

81. Erickson, H.K., Park, P.U., Widdison, W.C., et al. Antibody-maytansinoid conjugates are activated in targeted cancer cells by lysosomal degradation and linker-dependent intracellular processing. *Cancer Res.* 2006; 66 (8): 4426–33.

82. Saito, G., Swanson, J.A., Lee, K.D. Drug delivery strategy utilizing conjugation via reversible disulfide linkages: role and site of cellular reducing activities. *Adv. Drug Deliv. Rev.* 2003; 55 (2): 199–215.

83. Arner, E.S., Holmgren, A. Physiological functions of thioredoxin and thioredoxin reductase. *Eur. J. Biochem.* 2000; 267 (20): 6102–9.

84. Holmgren, A. Antioxidant function of thioredoxin and glutaredoxin systems. *Antioxid. Redox. Signal* 2000; 2 (4): 811–20.

85. Phan, U.T., Maric, M., Dick, T.P., Cresswell, P. Multiple species express thiol oxidoreductases related to GILT. *Immunogenetics* 2001; 53 (4): 342–6.

86. Phan, U.T., Arunachalam, B., Cresswell, P. Gamma-interferon-inducible lysosomal thiol reductase (GILT): maturation, activity, and mechanism of action. *J. Biol. Chem.* 2000; 275 (34): 25907–14.

87. Arunachalam, B., Phan, U.T., Geuze, H.J., Cresswell, P. Enzymatic reduction of disulfide bonds in lysosomes: characterization of a gamma-interferon-inducible lysosomal thiol reductase (GILT). *Proc. Natl. Acad. Sci. USA* 2000; 97 (2): 745–50.

88. Francisco, J.A., Cerveny, C.G., Meyer, D.L., et al. cAC10-vcMMAE, an anti-CD30-monomethyl auristatin E conjugate with potent and selective antitumor activity. *Blood* 2003; 102 (4): 1458–65.

89. Dubowchik, G.M., Firestone, R.A., Padilla, L., et al. Cathepsin B-labile dipeptide linkers for lysosomal release of doxorubicin from internalizing immunoconjugates: model studies of enzymatic drug release and antigen-specific in vitro anticancer activity. *Bioconjug. Chem.* 2002; 13 (4): 855–69.

90. Suzawa, T., Nagamura, S., Saito, H., Ohta, S., Hanai, N., Yamasaki, M. Synthesis of a novel duocarmycin derivative DU-257 and its application to immunoconjugate using poly(ethylene glycol)-dipeptidyl linker capable of tumor specific activation. *Bioorg. Med. Chem.* 2000; 8 (8): 2175–84.

91. de Groot, F.M., Albrecht, C., Koekkoek, R., Beusker, P.H., Scheeren, H.W. "Cascade-release dendrimers" liberate all end groups upon a single triggering event in the dendritic core. *Angew. Chem. Int. Ed. Engl.* 2003; 42 (37): 4490–4.

92. Freise, J., Muller, W.H., Brolsch, C., Schmidt, F.W. In vivo distribution of liposomes between parenchymal and non parenchymal cells in rat liver. *Biomedicine* 1980; 32 (3): 118–23.

93. Roerdink, F., Dijkstra, J., Hartman, G., Bolscher, B., Scherphof, G. The involvement of parenchymal, Kupffer and endothelial liver cells in the hepatic uptake of intrave-nously injected liposomes: effects of lanthanum and gadolinium salts. *Biochim. Bio-phys. Acta* 1981; 677 (1): 79–89.

94. Jones, M.N., Nicholas, A.R. The effect of blood serum on the size and stability of phospholipid liposomes. *Biochim. Biophys. Acta* 1991; 1065 (2): 145–52.

95. Schenkman, S., Araujo, P.S., Dijkman, R., Quina, F.H., Chaimovich, H. Effects of temperature and lipid composition on the serum albumin-induced aggregation and fusion of small unilamellar vesicles. *Biochim. Biophys. Acta* 1981; 649 (3): 633–47.

96. Hernandez-Caselles, T., Villalain, J., Gomez-Fernandez, J.C. Influence of liposome charge and composition on their interaction with human blood serum proteins. *Mol. Cell. Biochem.* 1993; 120 (2): 119–26.

97. Strejan, G.H., Essani, K., Surlan, D. Naturally occurring antibodies to liposomes, II: specificity and electrophoretic pattern of rabbit antibodies reacting with sphingomy-elin-containing liposomes. *J. Immunol.* 1981; 127 (1): 160–5.

98. Szebeni, J., Wassef, N.M., Rudolph, A.S., Alving, C.R. Complement activation in human serum by liposome-encapsulated hemoglobin: the role of natural anti-phospholipid antibodies. *Biochim. Biophys. Acta* 1996; 1285 (2): 127–30.

99. Klibanov, A.L., Maruyama, K., Torchilin, V.P., Huang, L. Amphipathic polyethylene-glycols effectively prolong the circulation time of liposomes. *FEBS Lett.* 1990; 268 (1): 235–7.

100. Blume, G., Cevc, G. Liposomes for the sustained drug release in vivo. *Biochim. Biophys. Acta* 1990; 1029 (1): 91–7.

101. Allen, T.M. The use of glycolipids and hydrophilic polymers in avoiding rapid uptake of liposomes by the mononuclear phagocyte system. *Adv. Drug Deliv. Rev.* 1994; 13 (3): 285–309.

102. Scherphof, G., Morselt, H., Allen, T. Intrahepatic distribution of long circulating liposomes containing poly (ethylene glycol) istearoyl phosphatidylethanolamine. *J. Liposome Res.* 1994; 4: 213–28.

103. Woodle, M.C., Storm, G., eds. *Long Circulating Liposomes: Old Drugs, New Therapeutics.* New York: Springer-Verlag; 1997.

104. Uziely, B., Jeffers, S., Isacson, R., et al. Liposomal doxorubicin: antitumor activity and unique toxicities during two complementary phase I studies. *J. Clin. Oncol.* 1995; 13 (7): 1777–85.

105. Maruyama, K., Takahashi, N., Tagawa, T., Nagaike, K., Iwatsuru, M. Immunoliposomes bearing polyethyleneglycol-coupled Fab' fragment show prolonged circulation time and high extravasation into targeted solid tumors in vivo. *FEBS Lett.* 1997; 413 (1): 177–80.

106. Moreira, J.N., Gaspar, R., Allen, T.M. Targeting Stealth liposomes in a murine model of human small cell lung cancer. *Biochim. Biophys. Acta* 2001; 1515 (2): 167–76.

107. Park, J.W., Kirpotin, D.B., Hong, K., et al. Tumor targeting using anti-HER2 immunoliposomes. *J. Control Release* 2001; 74 (1–3): 95–113.

108. Maruyama, K., Ishida, O., Takizawa, T., Moribe, K. Possibility of active targeting to tumor tissues with liposomes. *Adv. Drug Deliv. Rev.* 1999; 40 (1–2): 89–102.

109. Weinstein, J.N., van Osdol, W. Early intervention in cancer using monoclonal antibodies and other biological ligands: micropharmacology and the "binding site barrier." *Cancer Res.* 1992; 52 (9 Suppl.): 2747s–51s.

110. Park, J.W., Hong, K., Kirpotin, D.B., et al. Anti-HER2 immunoliposomes: enhanced efficacy attributable to targeted delivery. *Clin. Cancer Res.* 2002; 8 (4): 1172–81.

111. Lopes de Menezes, D.E., Pilarski, L.M., Allen, T.M. In vitro and in vivo targeting of immunoliposomal doxorubicin to human B-cell lymphoma. *Cancer Res.* 1998; 58 (15): 3320–30.

112. Sugano, M., Egilmez, N.K., Yokota, S.J., et al. Antibody targeting of doxorubicin-loaded liposomes suppresses the growth and metastatic spread of established human lung tumor xenografts in severe combined immunodeficient mice. *Cancer Res.* 2000; 60 (24): 6942–9.

113. Grillo-Lopez, A.J., Hedrick, E., Rashford, M., Benyunes, M. Rituximab: ongoing and future clinical development. *Semin. Oncol.* 2002; 29 (1 Suppl. 2): 105–12.

114. Leyland-Jones, B. Trastuzumab: hopes and realities. *Lancet Oncol.* 2002; 3 (3): 137–44.

115. Sievers, E.L., Linenberger, M. Mylotarg: antibody-targeted chemotherapy comes of age. *Curr. Opinion Oncol.* 2001; 13 (6): 522–7.

116. Ferrajoli, A., O'Brien, S., Keating, M.J. Alemtuzumab: a novel monoclonal antibody. *Expert Opinion Biol. Ther.* 2001; 1 (6): 1059–65.

117. Goldenberg, D.M. The role of radiolabeled antibodies in the treatment of non-Hodgkin's lymphoma: the coming of age of radioimmunotherapy. *Crit. Rev. Oncol. Hematol.* 2001; 39 (1–2): 195–201.

118. GlaxoSmithKline. Bexxar® for non-Hodgkin's Lymphoma. http://www.bexxar.com. Accessed March 4, 2007.

119. Genentech. Avastin® (bevacizumab). http://www.gene.com/gene/products/information/oncology/avastin. Accessed March 4, 2007.

120. Bristol-Meyers Squibb. Erbitux® (cetuximab). http://www.erbitux.com/erbitux/erb/home/index.jsp?BV_UseBVCookie=Yes. Accessed March 4, 2007.

121. Wahl, A.F., Donaldson, K.L., Mixan, B.J., Trail, P.A., Siegall, C.B. Selective tumor sensitization to taxanes with the mAb-drug conjugate cBR96-doxorubicin. *Int. J. Cancer* 2001; 93 (4): 590–600.

122. Mansfield, E., Pastan, I., FitzGerald, D.J. Characterization of RFB4-Pseudomonas exotoxin A immunotoxins targeted to CD22 on B-cell malignancies. *Bioconjug. Chem.* 1996; 7 (5): 557–63.

123. Johnson, T.A., Press, O.W. Therapy of B-cell lymphomas with monoclonal antibodies and radioimmunoconjugates: the Seattle experience. *Ann. Hematol.* 2000; 79 (4): 175–82.

124. Knox, S.J., Goris, M.L., Trisler, K., et al. Yttrium-90-labeled anti-CD20 monoclonal antibody therapy of recurrent B-cell lymphoma. *Clin. Cancer Res.* 1996; 2 (3): 457–70.

6 Relating Target Sequence to Biological Function

Greg M. Arndt

CONTENTS

INTRODUCTION

The completion of the human genome sequence has led to the need for functional annotation and determination of the roles of the newly identified genes in both normal cellular processes and disease states (1). A number of unexpected observations arose from the human genome sequence, including the lower number of predicted protein-coding genes and the fact that as many as three-quarters of these genes have no assigned biological function (2). The most surprising finding from this sequence was that only 2% of the genome encodes for proteins. By far the majority of the human transcriptome is composed of RNAs that do not code for proteins, the so-called noncoding RNA genes (3). The approaches used to discover novel genes and validate these sequences will require assessment of this unexpected gene population. Furthermore, the number of protein-coding genes without an assigned function has created a new bottleneck in drug discovery.

One of the most effective ways of identifying genes controlling complex cellular phenotypes and biological mechanisms of human disease is the use of chemical mutagenesis and forward genetic selections for modified phenotypes. For many years, this approach has been used in model organisms to identify key genes essential for specific phenotypic modifications (4). Chemical mutagenesis has only limited utility in mammalian cell systems and, as such, expression libraries have been used in combination with genetic selection (5, 6). Unlike differential gene expression analyses, screening of complex expression libraries for essential genes provides a functional link between the gene or genes and the cellular phenotype. Furthermore, identification of genes through phenotypic screening provides an immediate biological function to a newly identified sequence.

In this chapter, I review the principles of forward genetic selections in mammalian cell models for discovering the genes contributing to complex phenotypes associated with human disease. In addition, I discuss nucleic acid-based technology platforms for validating genes and confirming their biological roles. Throughout, the emphasis is on the need for an integrated approach to gene discovery involving both forward genetic (finding genes through phenotypes) and reverse genetic (validating the role of key genes essential to a phenotype) strategies to unravel the complexity of human disease and identify relevant target genes for drug discovery.

FORWARD GENETICS AND GENE DISCOVERY — PHENOTYPE TO GENE

Classical genetic approaches have been used in model organisms to determine the mechanisms responsible for gain or loss of gene functions. In general, this involves chemical mutagenesis of a starting population, identification of mutants displaying an altered phenotype, mapping the mutation by linkage analysis, positional cloning, and cloning of the genomic region containing the mutated gene. Besides being time consuming, the use of mutagenesis to induce mutations and perform forward genetic screens in mammalian cells has been restricted (6). Instead, the more common strategy for identifying genes involved in complex cellular processes has involved the combination of expression libraries, encoding trans-acting factors that modulate the expression of independent genes, with genetic screens designed to isolate rare cells displaying modified phenotypes. These can be caused by overexpression of genes (gain of function) or suppression of specific gene expression (loss of function). These forms of trans-dominant genetics are highly advantageous in organisms or cells that do not conform to traditional genetic manipulation, such as diploid or polyploid mammalian cell lines. Furthermore, the genetic agent responsible for the altered phenotype can be recovered and used to identify the key gene whose function is linked to that cellular modification.

The steps in using expression-library-based genetic selections in mammalian cells are outlined in Figure 6.1. This process involves the construction and characterization of the expression library, optimization of library delivery to the host cell population, selection for modified cellular phenotypes, recovery and characterization of library inserts, and identification of the genes implicated. The size and complexity

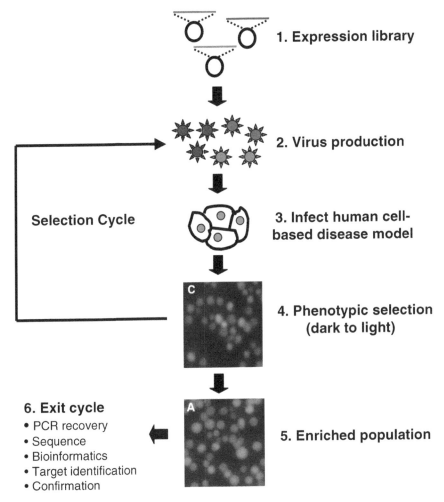

1. Expression library

2. Virus production

Selection Cycle

3. Infect human cell-based disease model

4. Phenotypic selection (dark to light)

6. Exit cycle
• PCR recovery
• Sequence
• Bioinformatics
• Target identification
• Confirmation

5. Enriched population

FIGURE 6.1 Using forward genetic selection in mammalian cells to discover novel genes. This schematic summarizes the process of forward genetic selections involving: (1) the generation of expression libraries; (2) production of virus containing individual members of the library; (3) delivery of the library to host cells by infection; (4) selection for cells displaying an altered cellular phenotype (e.g., dark to light); (5) continued cycles of selection to produce a cell population enriched for the modified phenotype (e.g., light); and (6) isolation of cells with the desired phenotype and characterization of the putative gene(s) involved.

of the expression library permits screening of a large number of target genes for their role in a particular cellular process. In addition, efficient methods of recovery of the library inserts from cells displaying the desired phenotype allow for multicycle selection to enrich the most relevant target genes and, ultimately, to identify those sequences. The platforms used for the genetic selections are flexible and can be performed using both biased and unbiased genetic-selection strategies. By defining the role of the genetic agent in modifying a cellular phenotype, one can identify

TABLE 6.1
Types of Expression Libraries
Used for Functional Gene
Screening in Mammalian Cells

Library Type	References
Single gene	23
Full-length cDNA	35
Antisense	21
Random fragment	44
Random sequence: ribozyme	18
Random sequence: peptide	19
RNAi	71

potential therapeutic targets and therapeutics (in the form of the agent) for manipulating phenotypes associated with human disease.

A number of different expression-library systems have been described for functional cloning of genes (Table 6.1). The vectors used for expression of the trans-acting genetic agents include episomal plasmids (7) and viruses, such as retroviral (8), lentiviral (9), and adenoviral vectors (10). Episomal plasmids are delivered by commonly used methods of DNA transfection, while viral vectors are transduced using recombinant viruses generated from packaging cell lines. The controlling elements for expression of the genetic agents are varied and include both constitutive and conditional promoters (11, 12). The sources of the inserts encoding the genetic agents include genomic DNA (13), cDNA (9), selected cDNAs (14), single genes (15, 16), and random oligonucleotides (17–19). The expression-library complexity varies from 1×10^5 to 1×10^8 different members, allowing for screening of a large genetic diversity. A number of different genetic markers are available to distinguish construct-bearing cells from cells lacking library members. These include selectable markers or drug-resistance genes, fluorescent protein genes, or fusion genes between genetic markers and the genetic agent (11).

The phenotypic bioassays used for forward genetic selections in mammalian cells must be sensitive and reflective of a key event or events in the disease process under investigation (Table 6.2). The optimal features of a genetic screen or bioassay that increase the probability of identifying relevant genetic agents include: predetermining the response of the host cell line to the desired stimulus or selection; efficient isolation of cells displaying the mutant phenotype; ensuring that cells showing this phenotype are not at a selective disadvantage; selecting host cells that are easily transfected or transduced with the highly complex library (>10^6 genetic agents); maximizing the expression level of the genetic agents; reducing the background of spontaneous mutants displaying the phenotype under consideration; and inclusion of methods for reducing false positives, such as multiple rounds of insert recovery and selection or exclusion of nontarget cell populations by the use of multiple parameters or conditional promoters (20). The most common genetic

TABLE 6.2
Cellular Phenotypes Useful in Forward Genetic Selection Strategies in Mammalian Cells

Gene/Protein Class	Selection/Screen
Cell-surface proteins	Flow cytometry
Extracellular proteins	Flow cytometry, proliferation, survival
Growth factors	Factor-dependent growth
Oncogenes	Loss of contact inhibition
Tumor suppressors	Tumorigenesis
Signaling proteins	Reporter activation
Transcription factors	Reporter activation
Apoptosis inhibitors	Resistance to apoptosis inducers
Metastasis-inducing genes	*In vitro* migration or invasion; *in vivo* metastasis to distant organs
Differentiation genes	Markers of differentiation
Cell-cycle proteins	Loss of contact inhibition; proliferation
Ion channels	Ion-specific indicators/tracers

screens involve a growth advantage for the cell containing a specific genetic agent, for example, resistance to a particular drug (19). Alternatively, flow cytometry can be used to identify and isolate rare cells displaying the desired phenotype (11). In most instances, multiple rounds of selection and amplification of inserts are required to enrich for the subset of genetic effectors directly contributing to the modified phenotype.

Upon isolation of the rare cells showing the mutant phenotype, the genetic effectors must be recovered and characterized. Methods for recovery of these agents include polymerase chain reaction (PCR) (14), plasmid isolation (21), delivery of packaging components to recover vector virus (22), and use of a site-specific recombination system (5). It is essential to reclone the effector insert and deliver it to the host cell population to confirm the link between expression of the genetic agent and the observed phenotype. Alternatively, inclusion of site-specific recombination sites flanking the genetic agent can be used to delete this sequence and determine whether the phenotype reverts (5). Recovery of the genetic agent allows for identification of the putative target gene. The methods for gene identification vary with the type of expression library used and include determination of the DNA sequence and homology searching.

Forward genetic selection is an extremely powerful technology for the identification of novel genes that regulate the essential pathways responsible for the onset and development of human disease. This approach results in both target identification and validation. The keys to the success of this strategy are highly complex genetic-expression libraries and sensitive biological assays that reflect essential features associated with the disease pathology. In the remainder of this section, I examine the range and diversity of gain-of-function and loss-of-function genetic screens and selections reported in mammalian cells.

GAIN-OF-FUNCTION SCREENS

Through the use of complex genetic-expression libraries it is possible to create new dominant cell phenotypes in mammalian cells by gene overexpression. Common examples of the kinds of traits that have been manipulated using this approach include resistance to drugs or stimuli, induction of tumorigenesis, and expression of surface markers. The end result of these genetic screens is a gain of function for the cell that is dependent on the introduced foreign DNA. Historically, this approach was first used to discover the activated Ha-ras oncogene from the T24 human bladder carcinoma cell line (13). In this study, genomic DNA isolated from these tumorigenic cells was transferred to mouse NIH 3T3 cells. Genetic selection was imposed to identify mouse cells displaying a tumorigenic phenotype, and the human genomic DNA was identified. The general principles of present-day forward genetics are reflected in this early study, i.e., using DNA from a mutant cell type as the "library," introducing this into nontumorigenic cells, and selecting for a gain of function in the form of tumorigenicity.

The simplest application of the gain-of-function selection strategy is the screening of single gene variants for new cellular functions or functional domains (Table 6.3). The basic strategy involves generating a variant-expression library by mutagenesis of the cDNA for the gene product under investigation. A variety of techniques can be used, including error-prone PCR (16) or DNA shuffling (23). These libraries are delivered to a host cell and subjected to genetic selection for cells expressing the gene product with newly acquired functional capabilities. Examples of these selection strategies include evolving T-cell receptor variants with altered binding affinities for viral epitopes (24), screening of scavenger receptor cDNA variants for those showing modified interactions with high-density and low-density lipoproteins (16), isolation of retroviruses with novel tropisms (25), and development of highly potent versions of cytokines (23).

In addition to single gene screens, complementation and dominant-effector studies have been performed in mammalian cells. Complementation involves the use of cDNA expression libraries to restore an original phenotype and, in turn, identify the gene or genes responsible for the mutant phenotype. Using Chinese hamster ovary (CHO) cells defective in cell-surface glycosylation, and therefore increased sensitivity to toxic lectins, Chatterton et al. (26) identified LDLB as a gene that corrects this defect by delivering a retroviral cDNA library and selecting for growth in the presence of ricin. Similar complementation screens have led to the identification of a novel protein required for folate import into the mitochondria (27), isolation of a human GDP-fucose transporter as the missing gene in patient cells deficient in protein glycosylation (28), and cloning of receptors for retroviruses and measles virus (29, 30).

In dominant-effector screens, cDNA expression libraries are scanned for cDNAs that, when overexpressed, result in a novel, dominant, and selectable phenotype. Through these kinds of genetic screens, it is possible to identify new genes that play roles in complex biological processes. Such functional genetic strategies have been used successfully to identify genes regulating apoptosis induced by different stimuli

TABLE 6.3
Examples of Gain-of-Function Genetic Screens Performed in Mammalian Cells

Strategy	Host Cells	Screen/Selection	References
Single gene variant	T-cell line	Influenza-specific TCR/FACS	24
	CHO	Scavenger receptor binding HDL/FACS	16
	Fibroblasts	MLV resistant to viral concentrating/infection assay	98
	CHO	Novel MLV tropism/viral infection assay	25
	COS7	Highly potent IL-12 cytokine/T-cell proliferation	23
Complementation	CHO	Correct glycosylation defect/growth in ricin	26
	CHO	Correct folate transport defect/ growth in absence of glycine	27
	Primary fibroblasts	Correct glycosylation defect/lectin staining assay	28
	CHO, NIH 3T3	Viral receptors/FACS or viral infection assays	29, 30
Dominant effectors	Mink lung epithelial	Overcome growth arrest by TGF-β/growth	34
	Jurkat T cells	Survival of Fas-induced apoptosis/growth	31
	Rat1/MycER fibroblasts	Overcome myc-induced apoptosis/growth	32
	NIH 3T3	*In vitro* transformation/foci formation	99
	Fibroblasts	Cytokine release/antigen presentation to T cells	36
	Mammary epithelial	Growth in the absence of EGF/growth	100
	SW480 colon cancer	Resistance to TRAIL-induced death/growth	33
	MEFs with T antigen	Bypass replicative senescence checkpoint/growth	35
	Jurkat T cells	Reduced TCR-activation-induced CD69/FACS	11
	Rat epithelial	Resistance to anoikis/attached growth	101
	CD4+ T cells	Resistance to cytopathic effects of HIV/survival	9
In vivo	Amelanotic A375P	Lung metastases/growth and microarray analysis	37
	Adenovirus+ MEFs	Induce tumorigenesis in immunocompetent mice/growth	38

Note: TCR, T-cell receptor; FACS, fluorescence-activated cell sorting; CHO, Chinese hamster ovary; HDL, high-density lipoprotein; MLV, murine leukemia virus; TGF, transforming growth factor; EGF, epidermal growth factor; TRAIL, TNF-related apoptosis-inducing ligand; HIV, human immunodeficiency virus.

(31–33), to isolate genes overcoming growth arrest (34) or bypassing replicative senescence (35), to identify tumor antigens (36), and to uncover novel signaling molecules for T-cell activation (11). Furthermore, functional expression cloning has been extended to *in vivo* genetic screens, particularly for identification of genes involved in metastasis of lowly metastatic cells in mice (37, 38).

LOSS-OF-FUNCTION SCREENS

Until very recently, the overexpression approach to gene discovery was somewhat limited to genetic selections leading to phenotypic changes that produced a positive functional outcome. In this regard, overexpression of any gene that induces cell-growth inhibition or cell death can be at a selective disadvantage, as cells containing this genetic effector would be lost from the cell population. To identify the role of these genes in cell processes, gene inactivation or silencing can be used, as loss of expression of these key genes would be expected to produce a functional output such as drug resistance, tumorigenesis, or expression of a selectable cell-surface protein. A wide variety of expression libraries encoding trans-acting dominant negative genetic effectors have been developed and used in mammalian cells to identify genes for which loss of function results in a novel trait. In this section, I review the most common forms of these libraries and highlight applications toward discovering new genes and assigning gene functions (Table 6.4).

Antisense Libraries

Antisense RNAs are complementary RNAs capable of hybridizing with a specific target mRNA to form double-stranded RNA, the latter of which can inhibit many steps in the pathway of gene expression (39). Antisense expression libraries can be constructed using a single gene and screened for the most effective antisense RNAs using phenotypic selection (15). In addition, antisense cDNA libraries can be constructed and used to generate a selectable phenotype for the discovery of new genes. For example, the Technical Knock Out (TKO) method has been used to identify death-promoting or proapoptotic genes (21). In this approach, an episomal-based antisense cDNA library was delivered to HeLa ovarian carcinoma cells normally sensitive to IFN-g-induced apoptosis. Selection for cell survival and growth following IFN-g treatment implicated five novel genes in cell death. Recently, this method has been extended to screening for cells more sensitive to apoptosis and identifying the key genes through loss of the resident episome due to cell death (7). This latter strategy allows for the identification of target genes that, upon silencing, result in the death of the host cells. These genes are ideal as therapeutic targets for elimination of tumor cells.

A modification of this approach has been reported for generating antisense RNA from endogenous gene loci, called the random homozygous knockout (RHKO) method (40). It involves using a construct containing a promoterless selectable marker with a conditional promoter upstream, and directed in the opposite direction to this marker, to randomly integrate into the host cell, such that each cell contains a single integration event. This population of cells is then induced for transcription

TABLE 6.4
Examples of Loss of Function Genetic Screens Performed in Mammalian Cells

Strategy	Host Cells	Screen/Selection	References
Antisense	Primary MEFs	Overcome p53-induced growth arrest/growth	15
	HeLa	Growth resistance to IFN-g/growth	21
	HeLa	Sensitivity to Fas-induced apoptosis/death and subtraction	7
	NIH 3T3	*In vitro* tumorigenesis/soft agar growth	40–43
Random fragment	REFs	*In vitro* transformation or etoposide resistance/growth	102
	Ovarian cancer A2780	Cisplatin resistance/growth	45
	HT1080 fibrosarcoma	Synthetic lethality/FACs	103
	NIH 3T3	Etoposide resistance/growth	44
	HT1080 fibrosarcoma	Resistance to amphidicolin/growth	48
	HL60, CEM-ss	Block productive and latent stages of HIV infection/FACs	50, 51
	CHO (GFP reporter)	Inhibit stress activation/FACS	104
	Mammary epithelial	*In vivo* tumorigenesis/growth	14
	HCT116 colon cancer	Induction of caspase 3 activity/FACS	12
	Rabies-sensitive cells	Inhibition of rabies replication/viral infection assay	105
	MDAMB231 breast cancer	Growth inhibition/cell survival	49
	CHO	Resistance to DNA damaging agent bleomycin/growth	46
	CHO	Resistance to topoisomerase II inhibitor/growth	47
	NIH 3T3	Protection from TNF-induced apoptosis/growth	106
Ribozyme	PA-1 ovarian carcinoma	Activation of BRCA1 promoter/reporter and FACS	17
	HeLa	IRES translation in HCV/reporter and growth	54
	HeLa	Anchorage-independent growth/soft-agar assay	53
	Fibroblasts	*In vitro* transformation/foci formation	112
	Neuroblastoma	Resistance to C2-ceramide-induced apoptosis/growth	107
	MCF7 breast cancer	Resistance to TNF-a and cycloheximide/growth	18
	HeLa (+ Fas receptor)	Delay or resistance to Fas-mediated apoptosis/survival	108
	HT1080 fibrosarcoma	Reduced chemotaxis/cell migration assay	55
	NIH 3T3	Cell migration and invasion/cell invasion assay	56

(continued on next page)

TABLE 6.4 (continued)
Examples of Loss of Function Genetic Screens Performed in Mammalian Cells

Strategy	Host Cells	Screen/Selection	References
	Myoblasts	Muscle differentiation/myoblast differentiation assay	58
	Melanoma	Lung metastasis/growth	59
Peptide	HeLa	Resistance to Taxol/growth	19
	B-cell hybridoma	MHC presentation/T-cell recognition	62
	HT1080 fibrosarcoma	Protease substrates/viral infection assay	109
	A549 lung tumor	Antiproliferation peptides/FACS and viral infection assay	63
RNAi	HeLa	Resistance to TRAIL-induced apoptosis/cell proliferation	110
	NIH 3T3	Proteasome function/reporter assay	71
	Primary fibroblasts	Overcome p53-dependent growth arrest/growth	72
	HEK 293T	Defects in cell-cycle control and cytokinesis/morphology	111
	HEK 293T	Regulation of NF-kB transcriptional activity/reporter	73

Note: IFN-g, interferon gamma; FACS, fluorescence-activated cell sorting; GFP, green fluorescent protein; TNF, tumor necrosis factor; IRES, internal ribosome entry site; HCV, hepatitis C virus; MHC, major histocompatibility complex.

from the antisense promoter to produce antisense RNA from the resident integration site. Phenotypic selection is then imposed, and cells displaying the modified trait are isolated and characterized for sequences flanking the site of integration to identify the gene involved. The conditional nature of the antisense promoter permits reversion of the modified phenotype by removal of the inducer for the promoter. This approach was used to identify a novel tumor suppressor called tsg101 that, upon inactivation, leads to cell transformation. RHKO has been used to identify other genes involved in neoplastic transformation and to produce tumor cell line models that undergo reversible tumorigenesis (41–43). A distinct advantage of the integrated antisense approach is the generation of a stable cell population that can be used for more than one form of forward genetic selection assay.

Random Fragment Libraries

An alternative expression-library approach involves the use of random fragments generated from a starting cDNA population (44). These inserts are cloned in the sense and antisense orientation and encode for RNA or truncated protein molecules that have the potential to block the activity of the target RNA or protein from which they were derived. Functional selection identifies biologically active genetic effectors, referred to as genetic suppression elements (GSEs), which can act through antisense RNA or through dominant-negative truncated proteins.

The GSE screening method has been used with single gene targets to identify the most accessible sites for antisense RNA, to map functional protein domains, and to identify effective peptide-based inhibitors of protein function (45). It has also been applied to whole cDNA populations for the identification of genes via functional selection. In this regard, the GSE strategy has been used to identify novel drug sensitivity genes or mechanisms of drug resistance (46–48), novel tumor-suppressor proteins (14), genes controlling cell growth (49), surface and secreted proteins essential for tumor cell survival (12), and GSEs from both host and viral genomes that specifically block induction of latent HIV and HIV replication (50, 51). Furthermore, this method is also conducive to *in vivo* genetic selection (14). An interesting outcome from the GSE selection for resistance to the replication inhibitor Aphidicolin was the requirement that GSEs to four different target genes achieve the resistance phenotype (48). This highlights the power of the forward genetic method for deciphering complex cellular phenotypes.

Random Sequence Libraries — Ribozyme

Ribozymes are small catalytic RNAs that have been used successfully to reduce the expression of a variety of cellular and viral targets (52). The most popular RNA catalytic motifs for the construction of random ribozyme libraries are the small domains, referred to as hairpin and hammerhead, isolated from small plant pathogens. Both hairpin and hammerhead ribozymes can be designed to bind to and cleave specific substrate RNAs by making the binding arms complementary to sequences flanking a GUC triplet in a specific target RNA.

Efforts have been made to use randomized sequences to construct hairpin or hammerhead ribozyme libraries by randomizing the binding arm sequences, thereby producing ribozymes capable of recognizing all GUC triplets (17, 18). Selection of ribozymes modifying cellular phenotypes can then be used to identify genes. The general strategy involves stably delivering a library of ribozyme genes to cells, with the aim of one ribozyme construct per cell; subjecting the cell population to phenotypic selection and isolating cells with the phenotype of interest; and recovering ribozyme genes and enriching for ribozymes targeting genes controlling this phenotype. Gene identification is based on the sequence of the ribozyme and the known complementarity between the binding arms (16 bases) and the target RNA (separated by a GUC triplet). The techniques to identify genes from ribozyme libraries include sequence homology searching, using the ribozyme as a primer in 5′ or 3′ RACE (rapid amplification of cDNA ends) or as a probe to screen cDNA libraries (17, 18).

Random ribozyme libraries have been used to identify: genes required for anchorage-independent growth (53), cofactors for IRES-mediated translation in the hepatitis C virus (54), regulators of oncogenes (BRCA1) (17), genes essential for cell migration and invasion and Fas- or TNF-induced apoptosis (18, 55–57), and myoblast differentiation genes (58). In addition, random hammerhead ribozyme libraries can be used to perform genetic selections *in vivo* (59).

Random Sequence Libraries — Peptide

Early peptide expression libraries in bacteria involved the fusion of the random peptides to carrier proteins that provide a scaffold and protect them from cellular proteases (60). To eliminate the need for a large carrier protein and to confer protease resistance to free peptides in mammalian cells, Xu et al. included the peptide sequence EFLIVIKS upstream and downstream of the random 18 amino acid peptide sequence (19). The advantage of a peptide expression library is that the expressed peptides interact with the protein targets and therefore have the potential to mimic the effects of small molecules on these same macromolecules. One possible disadvantage is the some-what cumbersome identification of the targets of these inhibitory peptides, which generally involves yeast two-hybrid screening. Alternatively, peptide analogs can be used as affinity reagents to isolate cellular interacting proteins (61).

Functionally active intracellular peptides and proteins have been discovered using randomized peptide expression libraries in combination with genetic selection assays. For example, peptide expression libraries have been used to define cellular responses and identify genes involved in complex cell processes, including identi-fication of: antigen peptides (62), inhibitors of Taxol-induced apoptosis (19), and regulators of the cell cycle (61, 63).

RNA Interference (RNAi) Expression Libraries

A recent addition to the armamentarium of gene silencing is the phenomenon of RNA interference, wherein double-stranded RNA can be used to inactivate gene expression by targeting degradation of homologous mRNA (64). This form of gene silencing was initially discovered in plants, and the mechanism of gene control was deciphered using *C. elegans* and Drosophila. In these latter studies, long double-stranded RNA (dsRNA) was shown to be cleaved into 21–24 base pair (bp) small interfering RNAs (siRNAs) that then act through association with a multiprotein complex, referred to as the RNA-induced silencing complex (RISC), to mediate targeted cleavage of complementary mRNAs (65). In mammalian cells, long dsRNA is less commonly used to induce silencing due to the presence of a global intracellular response system that recognizes the presence of these RNAs, represses protein synthesis, and activates turnover of mRNAs (66). Instead, RNAi-induced gene silenc-ing is accomplished using the 21-bp siRNAs (67). These can be delivered as synthetic dsRNAs or as small hairpin RNAs (shRNAs) expressed from RNA polymerase II or III promoters (68). A number of expression systems have been developed for shRNAs in mammalian cells, including plasmid, retroviral, lentiviral, and adenoviral vectors. In addition, other orientations of expression cassettes have been reported with the aim of generating two short, complementary RNAs that can hybridize to form functional siRNAs (69, 70).

The relative ease of designing effective siRNAs for RNAi in mammalian cells, and the development of a wide variety of gene-expressed methods, has resulted in widespread use of this gene-inactivation technology for gene identification and validation studies (64). To advance the utility of this technology for gene discovery, several groups have initiated the construction of genomewide RNAi libraries for use in functional studies in mammalian cells (71–73). This strategy has been used with great effectiveness in model organisms (74). For each mouse or human gene, three different shRNA-expression cassettes are being constructed in retroviral-based vec-tors. In addition, sequence identifiers, or barcodes, are being included to permit tracking of different gene constructs (71, 72). This coding system permits the use of these libraries in different formats for gene discovery. In the arrayed format, each expression vector is deposited in a separate spot or well, and reverse transfection is used to deliver the DNA to the host cells. Each transfected cell population is then examined for phenotypic changes. With the barcoding system, the genomewide RNAi libraries can also be used in unbiased genetic selection formats, as discussed earlier. In this strategy, the libraries are delivered en masse, and a pooled population is subjected to functional selection to isolate rare cells displaying an altered phenotype due to RNAi-mediated loss of function of a specific gene target. These libraries have been used to characterize components of the human proteasome and to identify novel modulators of p53-dependent growth arrest (71, 72). It is anticipated that these reagents will be used for further mammalian cell functional screens both in culture and *in vivo*.

An exciting application of the barcoded genomewide RNAi libraries in mammalian cells is the opportunity to perform synthetic lethality genetic selections. Two mutations are synthetically lethal if cells with either of the single mutations are viable but cells with both mutations are nonviable. In many cancers, the genetic changes that exist within cells at different stages of tumor development have been identified. Using RNAi libraries, it is possible to isolate genes that, upon loss of function in genetically defined cancer cells, result in a growth disadvantage or death (75). Normally these cells are lost from the population, and identification of the genes responsible for these phenotypes is difficult. However, by creating a DNA microarray containing all of the barcodes for the RNAi library, it is possible to monitor the relative abundance of each construct in the population by harvesting DNA, labeling it with a fluorescent dye, and then hybridizing to the array. Any cells showing slower growth or undergoing cell death lose the resident library inserts. This will be reflected in a weaker signal on the array (76). A similar approach, called selection subtraction, combines functional genetic selection with molecular screening to identify key genes (77).

VALIDATING NOVEL GENES — GENE TO PHENOTYPE

As indicated earlier, forward genetic selections both identify and validate genes. However, utilization of an alternative technique to control the expression of a specific gene and reproduce the associated phenotype increases confidence in the potential target for drug development. Furthermore, the development of high-throughput technologies for biology have led to the generation of lists of genes with an association with the disease state, but with no direct functional evidence for a link. Reverse genetics assesses or confirms whether a gene is involved in a specific cellular phenotype. In general, this involves regulating the expression of a specific gene, either through overexpression or suppression, and then testing whether changes in the level of the gene product affect disease-related phenotypes. A number of technology platforms have been developed for gene silencing in mammalian cells. The current methods are designed to target DNA, RNA, or protein, with the aim of blocking the function of the gene at different levels of the gene-expression pathway.

TABLE 6.5
Gene-Silencing Technologies

Feature	Ribozymes	DNAzymes	EGS	RNAi
Mode of action	Artificial	Artificial	Natural	Natural
Specificity	Lingering questions	Lingering questions	High	High
"Universality"	Low	Low	Low	High
Use range *in vitro*	Low µM to high nM	Low µM to high nM	Low µM to high nM	Low nM
Site selection	Systematic	Systematic	Systematic	Algorithms; systematic
Range of targets	Moderate to wide	Moderate	Moderate	Wide
	Cellular and viral	Cellular	Cellular and viral	Cellular and viral
Off-target effects	Yes	Unknown	Unknown	Yes; controversial
Side effects	Protein binding	Unknown	Unknown	IFN response
Subcellular site	Nucleus and cytoplasm	Nucleus and cytoplasm	Nucleus	Nucleus and cytoplasm
Modalities	Synthetic; gene-express	Synthetic	Synthetic; gene-express	Synthetic; gene-express
Major strengths	Simple catalytic domain	Inexpensive	Natural mechanism	Effective at low levels
	Target introns	Good *in vitro* catalysis	Flexibility in design	Multiple mechanisms
	Tissue-specific expression			Tissue-specific expression
Major weaknesses	Requires GUC triplet	Off-target effects?	Too few studies	No option for refractory target
	Possible aptamer activity	Synthetic only		Possible off-target effects

This section focuses on the key technologies using nucleic acids to induce transcriptional or posttranscriptional gene silencing and their utility in reverse genetics
(Table 6.5) (78).

RIBOZYMES

The observation that RNA could catalyze the cleavage and ligation of RNA led to
the development of small catalytic RNAs, or ribozymes, for use as tools for gene
silencing and as potential therapeutics (52). To date, the most popular ribozyme motif
is the hammerhead ribozyme, originally identified from the small plant pathogenic
RNA associated with the tobacco ringspot virus. The standard design for these
ribozymes includes two binding arms (of seven to nine nucleotides) complementary
to the target RNA, flanking any UH sequence (where H is U, C, or A), and separated
by a 21-base catalytic core domain. Through Watson–Crick base pairing, the hammerhead ribozyme recognizes target RNA and mediates cleavage to produce products
having 2′–3′ cyclic phosphate and 5′-hydroxyl termini. The ribozyme sequence can

be delivered as a synthetic RNA or expressed from a variety of different promoters in a wide range of mammalian cell types. The limitations of this technology are the requirement for a specific triplet codon at the cleavage site in the target RNA and the propensity for ribozymes to bind cellular proteins (52, 79). These trans-acting catalytic RNAs have been used to target many different classes of genes and associated gene products as well as viral targets associated with infectious disease (80).

DNAzymes

DNAzymes are small catalytic DNAs capable of hybridizing to complementary RNAs and mediating specific cleavage to generate end products similar to those produced by hammerhead ribozyme-directed cleavage (81). As with ribozymes, these catalytic DNAs have the potential to recycle and direct cleavage of multiple target RNAs. The common DNAzyme catalytic motifs were evolved by *in vitro* selection (82), and application of these DNAzymes for *in vitro* diagnostics has been very successful (83). There have been several reports on the use of these catalytic DNAs to control specific gene expression in cell culture and in animals (81). At present, DNAzymes are delivered as synthetic DNA molecules, although recent development of single-stranded DNA vectors for mammalian cells may provide the vehicle for intracellular generation of these sequences (84).

External Guide Sequences (EGSs)

The development of EGS technology for silencing gene expression stemmed from the characterization of RNase-P-mediated cleavage of pre-tRNA molecules to produce mature tRNAs (85). These studies identified RNA as the catalytic component of the RNase P ribonucleoprotein complex. Moreover, characterization of the substrate showed that the structure recognized by RNase P could be mimicked using antisense RNAs, called EGSs, which hybridize with any target RNA and reproduce a tRNA-like structure. EGSs can be synthetic or gene-expressed and have been used primarily to target mammalian viruses, including herpes simplex virus (HSV), cytomegalovirus (CMV), and human immunodeficiency virus (HIV) (86, 87). As with all gene-silencing technologies operating at the posttranscriptional level, the identification of target RNA sites accessible to EGS binding is essential for efficient control of gene expression. One advantage associated with EGSs for gene silencing is its action through a naturally occurring cellular machinery that has evolved to cleave and modify small RNAs.

RNAi

The discovery that dsRNA could act as a potent and specific mediator of gene silencing has led to a revolution in the use of RNAi to determine the function of genes and to identify potential drug targets in mammalian cells (64). Based on an understanding of the RNAi mechanism and testing of multiple synthetic siRNAs as well as gene-expressed shRNAs to several target RNAs, design rules and associated algorithms have been developed for identifying potential RNAi-sensitive sites on target RNA (88, 89). In most instances, systematic analysis of three different siRNAs, or shRNAs, per target identified an effective gene-silencing agent that reduces target RNA levels by between 50 and 70%. A variety of methods can be used for the delivery of synthetic siRNAs, and several different vector systems exist for expression of shRNAs in mammalian cells (68, 90). This form of gene silencing has been applied to a range of different molecular and biological targets, most of which have been exhaustively reviewed (68). One potentially attractive feature of RNAi for gene functional studies is the capacity to generate an epi-allelic series of cell clones for a specific target gene using shRNA-expression vectors (91). In addition, the ability to express shRNAs that undergo processing to direct RNAi-mediated gene silencing of specific target RNAs has inspired the development and testing of longer dsRNAs in mammalian cells, with the aim of producing multiple siRNA products (92). Theoretically, these multidomain dsRNA hairpins could be used to produce multiple siRNAs to a single target or to generate single siRNAs to many different targets. The current limitations with RNAi are the potential for off-target effects and induction of the interferon response due to the promiscuous nature of RNA-mediated gene silencing for some target sites (see (93) for comment). This remains controversial and will require further experimental studies.

An exciting extension of posttranscriptional silencing by siRNAs is the potential for inducing sequence-specific transcriptional silencing using the RNAi machinery (94). RNAi-mediated DNA methylation and associated transcriptional silencing was first demonstrated in plants (95). More recently, two independent studies have shown that synthetic siRNAs or gene-expressed shRNAs directed against mammalian promoters, and localized to the cell nucleus, could induce DNA methylation at their associated target sites in the genome (96, 97). This approach to gene silencing in mammalian cells may provide an alternative route for inactivating specific gene expression at the level of the gene itself.

CONCLUDING REMARKS

The pathology of human disease is directed by alterations to the interplay and coordinated regulation of multiple genes, the end result of which is the generation of a "mutant" (or disease) phenotype. Deciphering this complexity, and understanding the underlying biological mechanisms, requires an integrated approach. Using forward genetic selection, changes in the cellular phenotypes related to the disease condition drives the identification of genes essential to the biological process, directly linking cellular targets to the cellular phenotype. In addition, it pinpoints particular cell-signaling pathways and networks that control cellular responses in human disease. Combining this information with other technologies, such as subtractive hybridization or differential gene expression analyses, provides an integrated platform for gene discovery. Genes identified as either linked to a particular cellular response or associated with this response can be further examined for gene function using reverse genetic strategies, such as the wide array of gene-silencing tools available for use in mammalian cells. It is this integration of forward genetics (to identify genes or groups of genes) with reverse genetics and creative cell biology (to decipher the precise role of those genes) that will provide a pathway toward relating target sequence to biological function.

REFERENCES

1. Smith, C. Drug target validation — hitting the target. *Nature* 2004; 422: 341–351.
2. Mattick, J.S. The human genome and the future of medicine. *Medical J. Australia* 2003; 179: 212–216.
3. Morey, C., Avner, P. Employment opportunities for non-coding RNAs. *FEBS Lett.* 2004; 567: 27–34.
4. David, R.H. The age of model organisms. *Nat. Rev. Genet.* 2004; 5: 69–76.
5. Hannon, G.J., Sun, P., Carnero, A., Xie, L.Y., Maestro, R., Conklin, D.S., Beach, D. MaRX: an approach to genetics in mammalian cells. *Science* 1999; 283: 1129–1130.
6. Stark, G.R., Gudkov, A.V. Forward genetics in mammalian cells: functional approaches to gene discovery. *Hum. Mol. Genet.* 1999; 8: 1925–1938.
7. Kotlo, K.U., Yehiely, F., Efimova, E., Harasty, H., Hesabi, B., Shchors, K., Einat, P., Rozen, A., Berent, E., Deiss, L.P. Nrf2 is an inhibitor of the Fas pathway as identified by Achilles' Heel Method, a new function-based approach to gene identification in human cells. *Oncogene* 2003; 22: 797–806.
8. Lorens, J.B., Sousa, C., Bennett, M.K., Molineaux, S.M., Payan, D.G. The use of retroviruses as pharmaceutical tools for target discovery and validation in the field of functional genomics. *Curr. Opin. Biotech.* 2001; 12: 613–621.
9. Kawano, Y., Yoshida, T., Hieda, K., Aoki, J., Miyoshi, H., Koyanagi, Y. A lentiviral cDNA library employing lambda recombination used to clone an inhibitor of human immunodeficiency virus type 1-induced cell death. *J. Virol.* 2004; 78: 11352–11359.
10. McVey, D., Zuber, M., Brough, D.E., Kovesdi, I. Adenovirus vector library: an approach to the discovery of gene and protein function. *J. Gen. Virol.* 2003; 84: 3417–3422.
11. Chu, P., Pardo, J., Zhao, H., Li, C.C., Pali, E., Shen, M.M., Qu, K., Yu, S.X., Huang, B.C., Yu, P., Masuda, E.S., Molineaux, S.M., Kolbinger, F., Aversa, G., de Vries, J., Payan, D.G., Liao, X.C. Systematic identification of regulatory proteins critical for T-cell activation. *J. Biol.* 2003; 2: 21.
12. Gelman, M.S., Ye, X.K., Stull, R., Suhy, D., Jin, L., Ng, D., Than, B., Ji, M., Pan, A., Perez, P., Sun, Y., Yeung, P., Garcia, L.M., Harte, R., Lu, Y., Lamar, E., Tavassoli, R., Kennedy, S., Osborn, S., Chin, D.J., Meshaw, K., Holzmayer, T.A., Axenovich, S.A., Abo, A. Identification of cell surface and secreted proteins essential for tumor cell survival using a genetic suppressor element screen. *Oncogene* 2004; 23: 8158–8170.
13. Goldfarb, M., Shimizu, K., Perucho, M., Wigler, M. Isolation and preliminary characterization of a human transforming gene from T24 bladder carcinoma cells. *Nature* 1982; 296: 404–409.
14. Garkavtsev, I., Kazarov, A., Gudkov, A., Riabowol, K. Suppression of the novel growth inhibitor p33ING1 promotes neoplastic transformation. *Nat. Genet.* 1996; 14: 415–420.
15. Carnero, A., Hudson, J.D., Hannon, G.J., Beach, D.H. Loss-of-function genetics in mammalian cells: the p53 tumor suppressor model. *Nucleic Acids Res.* 2000; 28: 2234–2241.
16. Gu, X., Lawrence, R., Krieger, M. Dissociation of the high-density lipoprotein and low density lipoprotein binding activities of murine scavenger receptor class B type I (mSR-BI) using retrovirus library-based activity dissection. *J. Biol. Chem.* 2000; 275: 9120–9130.
17. Beger, C., Pierce, L.N., Kruger, M., Marcusson, E.G., Robbins, J.M., Welcsh, P., Welch, P.J., Welte, K., King, M.C., Barber, J.R., Wong-Staal, F. Identification of Id4 as a regulator of BRCA1 expression by using a ribozyme-library-based inverse genomics approach. *Proc. Natl. Acad. Sci. USA* 2001; 98: 130–135.

18. Kawasaki, H., Onuki, R., Suyama, E., Taira, K. Identification of genes that function in the TNF-alpha-mediated apoptotic pathway using randomized hybrid ribozyme libraries. *Nat. Biotechnol.* 2002; 20: 376–380.

19. Xu, X., Leo, C., Jang, Y., Chan, E., Padilla, D., Huang, B.C., Lin, T., Gururaja, T., Hitoshi, Y., Lorens, J.B., Anderson, D.C., Sikic, B., Luo, Y., Payan, D.G., Nolan, G.P. Dominant effector genetics in mammalian cells. *Nat. Genet.* 2001; 27: 23–29.

20. Richards, B., Karpilow, J., Dunn, C., Zharkikh, L., Maxfield, A., Kamb, A., Teng, D.H. Creation of a stable human reporter cell line suitable for FACS-based, transdominant genetic selection. *Somat. Cell Mol. Genet.* 1999; 25: 191–205.

21. Deiss, L.P., Kimchi, A. A genetic tool used to identify thioredoxin as a mediator of a growth inhibitory signal. *Science* 1991; 252: 117–120.

22. Bhattacharya, D., Logue, E.C., Bakkour, S., DeGregori, J., Sha, W.C. Identification of gene function by cyclical packaging rescue of retroviral cDNA libraries. *Proc. Natl. Acad. Sci. USA* 2002; 99: 8838–8843.

23. Leong, S.R., Chang, J.C., Ong, R., Dawes, G., Stemmer, W.P., Punnonen, J. Optimized expression and specific activity of IL-12 by directed molecular evolution. *Proc. Natl. Acad. Sci. USA* 2003; 100: 1163–1168.

24. Kessels, H.W., van Den Boom, M.D., Spits, H., Hooijberg, E., Schumacher, T.N. Changing T cell specificity by retroviral T cell receptor display. *Proc. Natl. Acad. Sci. USA* 2000; 97: 14578–14583.

25. Soong, N.W., Nomura, L., Pekrun, K., Reed, M., Sheppard, L., Dawes, G., Stemmer, W.P. Molecular breeding of viruses. *Nat. Genet.* 2000; 25: 436–439.

26. Chatterton, J.E., Hirsch, D., Schwartz, J.J., Bickel, P.E., Rosenberg, R.D., Lodish, H.F., Krieger, M. Expression cloning of LDLB, a gene essential for normal Golgi function and assembly of the ldlCp complex. *Proc. Natl. Acad. Sci. USA* 1999; 96: 915–920.

27. Titus, S.A., Moran, R.G. Retrovirally mediated complementation of the glyB phenotype: cloning of a human gene encoding the carrier for entry of folates into mitochondria. *J. Biol. Chem.* 2000; 275: 36811–36817.

28. Lubke, T., Marquardt, T., Etzioni, A., Hartmann, E., von Figura, K., Korner, C. Complementation cloning identifies CDG-IIc, a new type of congenital disorders of glycosylation, as a GDP-fucose transporter deficiency. *Nat. Genet.* 2001; 28: 73–76.

29. Tailor, C.S., Nouri, A., Lee, C.G., Kozak, C., Kabat, D. Cloning and characterization of a cell surface receptor for xenotropic and polytropic murine leukemia viruses. *Proc. Natl. Acad. Sci. USA* 1999; 96: 927–932.

30. Erlenhoefer, C., Wurzer, W.J., Loffler, S., Schneider-Schaulies, S., ter Meulen, V., Schneider-Schaulies, J. CD150 (SLAM) is a receptor for measles virus but is not involved in viral contact-mediated proliferation inhibition. *J. Virol.* 2001; 75: 4499–4505.

31. Hitoshi, Y., Lorens, J., Kitada, S.I., Fisher, J., LaBarge, M., Ring, H.Z., Francke, U., Reed, J.C., Kinoshita, S., Nolan, G.P. Toso, a cell surface, specific regulator of Fas-induced apoptosis in T cells. *Immunity* 1998; 8: 461–471.

32. Maestro, R., Dei Tos, A.P., Hamamori, Y., Krasnokutsky, S., Sartorelli, V., Kedes, L., Doglioni, C., Beach, D.H., Hannon, G.J. Twist is a potential oncogene that inhibits apoptosis. *Genes Dev.* 1999; 13: 2207–2217.

33. Burns, T.F., El-Deiry, W.S. Identification of inhibitors of TRAIL-induced death (ITIDs) in the TRAIL-sensitive colon carcinoma cell line SW480 using a genetic approach. *J. Biol. Chem.* 2001; 276: 37879–37886.

34. Sun, P., Dong, P., Dai, K., Hannon, G.J., Beach, D. p53-Independent role of MDM2 in TGF-beta1 resistance. *Science* 1998; 282: 2270–2272.

35. Shvarts, A., Brummelkamp, T.R., Scheeren, F., Koh, E., Daley, G.Q., Spits, H., Bernards, R. A senescence rescue screen identifies BCL6 as an inhibitor of anti-proliferative p19(ARF)-p53 signaling. *Genes Dev.* 2002; 16: 681–686.

36. Wang, R.F., Wang, X., Johnston, S.L., Zeng, G., Robbins, P.F., Rosenberg, S.A. Development of a retrovirus-based complementary DNA expression system for the cloning of tumor antigens. *Cancer Res.* 1998; 58: 3519–3525.

37. Clark, E.A., Golub, T.R., Lander, E.S., Hynes, R.O. Genomic analysis of metastasis reveals an essential role for RhoC. *Nature* 2000; 406: 532–535.

38. Edel, M.J., Shvarts, A., Medema, J.P., Bernards, R. An in vivo functional genetic screen reveals a role for the TRK-T3 oncogene in tumor progression. *Oncogene* 2004; 23: 4959–4965.

39. Brantl, S. Antisense-RNA regulation and RNA interference. *Biochim. Biophys. Acta* 2002; 1575: 15–25.

40. Li, L., Cohen, S.N. Tsg101: a novel tumor susceptibility gene isolated by controlled homozygous functional knockout of allelic loci in mammalian cells. *Cell* 1996; 85: 319–329.

41. Liu, K., Li, L., Nisson, P.E., Gruber, C., Jessee, J., Cohen, S.N. Reversible tumori-genesis induced by deficiency of vasodilator-stimulated phosphoprotein. *Mol. Cell Biol.* 1999; 19: 3696–3703.

42. Liu, K., Li, L., Nisson, P.E., Gruber, C., Jessee, J., Cohen, S.N. Neoplastic transfor-mation and tumorigenesis associated with sam68 protein deficiency in cultured murine fibroblasts. *J. Biol. Chem.* 2000; 275: 40195–40201.

43. Liu, K., Li, L., Cohen, S.N. Antisense RNA-mediated deficiency of the calpain protease, nCL-4, in NIH3T3 cells is associated with neoplastic transformation and tumorigenesis. *J. Biol. Chem.* 2000; 275: 31093–31098.

44. Gudkov, A.V., Kazarov, A.R., Thimmapaya, R., Axenovich, S.A., Mazo, I.A., Ron-inson, I.B. Cloning mammalian genes by expression selection of genetic suppressor elements: association of kinesin with drug resistance and cell immortalization. *Proc. Natl. Acad. Sci. USA* 1994; 91: 3744–3748.

45. Gallagher, W.M., Cairney, M., Schott, B., Roninson, I.B., Brown, R. Identification of p53 genetic suppressor elements which confer resistance to cisplatin. *Oncogene* 1997; 14: 185–193.

46. Sanz, G., Mir, L., Jacquemin-Sablon, A. Bleomycin resistance in mammalian cells expressing a genetic suppressor element derived from the SRPK1 gene. *Cancer Res.* 2002; 62: 4453–4458.

47. Gros, L., Delaporte, C., Frey, S., Decesse, J., de Saint-Vincent, B.R., Cavarec, L., Dubart, A., Gudkov, A.V., Jacquemin-Sablon, A. Identification of new drug sensitivity genes using genetic suppressor elements: protein arginine N-methyltransferase medi-ates cell sensitivity to DNA-damaging agents. *Cancer Res.* 2003; 63: 164–171.

48. Levenson, V.V., Lausch, E., Kirschling, D.J., Broude, E.V., Davidovich, I.A., Libants, S., Fedosova, V., Roninson, I.B. A combination of genetic suppressor elements produces resistance to drugs inhibiting DNA replication. *Somat. Cell Mol. Genet.* 1999; 25: 9–26.

49. Primiano, T., Baig, M., Maliyekkel, A., Chang, B.D., Fellars, S., Sadhu, J., Axenovich, S.A., Holzmayer, T.A., Roninson, I.B. Identification of potential anticancer drug targets through the selection of growth-inhibitory genetic suppressor elements. *Can-cer Cell* 2003; 4: 41–53.

50. Dunn, S.J., Park, S.W., Sharma, V., Raghu, G., Simone, J.M., Tavassoli, R., Young, L.M., Ortega, M.A., Pan, C.H., Alegre, G.J., Roninson, I.B., Lipkina, G., Dayn, A., Holzmayer, T.A. Isolation of efficient antivirals: genetic suppressor elements against HIV-1. *Gene Ther.* 1999; 6: 130–137.

51. Dunn, S.J., Khan, I.H., Chan, U.A., Scearce, R.L., Melara, C.L., Paul, A.M., Sharma, V., Bih, F.Y., Holzmayer, T.A., Luciw, P.A., Abo, A. Identification of cell surface targets for HIV-1 therapeutics using genetic screens. *Virology* 2004; 321: 260–273.

52. Khan, A.U., Lal, S.K. Ribozymes: a modern tool in medicine. *J. Biomed. Sci.* 2003; 10: 457–467.

53. Welch, P.J., Marcusson, E.G., Li, Q.X., Beger, C., Kruger, M., Zhou, C., Leavitt, M., Wong-Staal, F., Barber, J.R. Identification and validation of a gene involved in anchorage-independent cell growth control using a library of randomized hairpin ribozymes. *Genomics* 2000; 66: 274–283.

54. Kruger, M., Beger, C., Li, Q.X., Welch, P.J., Tritz, R., Leavitt, M., Barber, J.R., Wong-Staal, F., Identification of eIF2Bgamma and eIF2gamma as cofactors of hepatitis C virus internal ribosome entry site-mediated translation using a functional genomics approach. *Proc. Natl. Acad. Sci. USA* 2000; 97: 8566–8571.

55. Suyama, E., Kawasaki, H., Kasaoka, T., Taira, K. Identification of genes responsible for cell migration by a library of randomized ribozymes. *Cancer Res.* 2003; 63: 119–124.

56. Suyama, E., Kawasaki, H., Nakajima, M., Taira, K. Identification of genes involved in cell invasion by using a library of randomized hybrid ribozymes. *Proc. Natl. Acad. Sci. USA* 2003; 100: 5616–5621.

57. Kawasaki, H., Taira, K. A functional gene discovery in the Fas-mediated pathway to apoptosis by analysis of transiently expressed randomized hybrid-ribozyme libraries. *Nucleic Acids Res.* 2002; 30: 3609–3614.

58. Wadhwa, R., Yaguchi, T., Kaur, K., Suyama, E., Kawasaki, H., Taira, K., Kaul, S.C. Use of a randomized hybrid ribozyme library for identification of genes involved in muscle differentiation. *J. Biol. Chem.* 2004; 279: 51622–51629.

59. Suyama, E., Wadhwa, R., Kaur, K., Miyagishi, M., Kaul, S.C., Kawasaki, H., Taira, K. Identification of metastasis-related genes in a mouse model using a library of randomized ribozymes. *J. Biol. Chem.* 2004; 279: 38083–38086.

60. Blum, J.H., Dove, S.L., Hochschild, A., Mekalanos, J.J. Isolation of peptide aptamers that inhibit intracellular processes. *Proc. Natl. Acad. Sci. USA* 2000; 97: 2241–2246.

61. Gururaja, T., Li, W., Catalano, S., Bogenberger, J., Zheng, J., Keller, B., Vialard, J., Janicot, M., Li, L., Hitoshi, Y., Payan, D.G., Anderson, D.C. Cellular interacting proteins of functional screen-derived antiproliferative and cytotoxic peptides discovered using shotgun peptide sequencing. *Chem. Biol.* 2003; 10: 927–937.

62. Tolstrup, A.B., Duch, M., Dalum, I., Pedersen, F.S., Mouritsen, S. Functional screening of a retroviral peptide library for MHC class I presentation. *Gene* 2001; 263: 77–84.

63. Hitoshi, Y., Gururaja, T., Pearsall, D.M., Lang, W., Sharma, P., Huang, B., Catalano, S.M., McLaughlin, J., Pali, E., Peelle, B., Vialard, J., Janicot, M., Wouters, W., Luyten, W., Bennett, M.K., Anderson, D.C., Payan, D.G., Lorens, J.B., Bogenberger, J., Demo, S. Cellular localization and antiproliferative effect of peptides discovered from a functional screen of a retrovirally delivered random peptide library. *Chem. Biol.* 2003; 10: 975–987.

64. Hannon, G.J., Rossi, J.J. Unlocking the potential of the human genome with RNA interference. *Nature* 2004; 431: 371–378.

65. Meister, G., Tuschl, T. Mechanisms of gene silencing by double-stranded RNA. *Nature* 2004; 431: 343–349.

66. Wang, Q., Carmichael, G.G. Effects of length and location on the cellular response to double-stranded RNA. *Microbiol. Mol. Biol. Rev.* 2004; 68: 432–452.

67. Dorsett, Y., Tuschl, T. siRNAs: Applications in functional genomics and potential as therapeutics. *Nat. Rev. Drug Discov.* 2004; 3: 318–329.

68. Dykxhoorn, D.M., Novina, C.D., Sharp, P.A. Killing the messenger: short RNAs that silence gene expression. *Nat. Rev. Mol. Cell Biol.* 2003; 4: 457–467.

69. Lee, N.S., Dohjima, T., Bauer, G., Li, H., Li, M.J., Ehsani, A., Salvaterra, P., Rossi, J. Expression of small interfering RNAs targeted against HIV-1 rev transcripts in human cells. *Nat. Biotechnol.* 2002; 20: 500–505.

70. Tran, N., Cairns, M.J., Dawes, I.W., Arndt, G.M. Expressing functional siRNAs in mammalian cells using convergent transcription. *BMC Biotechnol.* 2003; 3: 21.

71. Paddison, P.J., Silva, J.M., Conklin, D.S., Schlabach, M., Li, M., Aruleba, S., Balija, V., O'Shaughnessy, A., Gnoj, L., Scobie, K., Chang, K., Westbrook, T., Cleary, M., Sachidanandam, R., McCombie, W.R., Elledge, S.J., Hannon, G.J. A resource for large-scale RNA-interference-based screens in mammals. *Nature* 2004; 428: 427–431.

72. Berns, K., Hijmans, E.M., Mullenders, J., Brummelkamp, T.R., Velds, A., Heimerikx, M., Kerkhoven, R.M., Madiredjo, M., Nijkamp, W., Weigelt, B., Agami, R., Ge, W., Cavet, G., Linsley, P.S., Beijersbergen, R.L., Bernards, R. A large-scale RNAi screen in human cells identifies new components of the p53 pathway. *Nature* 2004; 428: 431–437.

73. Zheng, L., Liu, J., Batalov, S., Zhou, D., Orth, A., Ding, S., Schultz, P.G. An approach to genomewide screens of expressed small interfering RNAs in mammalian cells. *Proc. Natl. Acad. Sci. USA* 2004; 101: 135–140.

74. Nollen, E.A., Garcia, S.M., van Haaften, G., Kim, S., Chavez, A., Morimoto, R.I., Plasterk, R.H. Genome-wide RNA interference screen identifies previously undescribed regulators of polyglutamine aggregation. *Proc. Natl. Acad. Sci. USA* 2004; 101: 6403–6408.

75. Garber, K. Running interference: pace picks up on synthetic lethality research. *J. Natl. Cancer Inst.* 2004; 96: 982–983.

76. Brummelkamp, T.R., Bernards, R. New tools for functional mammalian cancer genetics. *Nat. Rev. Cancer* 2003; 3: 781–789.

77. Singhi, A.D., Kondratov, R.V., Neznanov, N., Chernov, M.V., Gudkov, A.V. Selection-subtraction approach (SSA): a universal genetic screening technique that enables negative selection. *Proc. Natl. Acad. Sci. USA* 2004; 101: 9327–9332.

78. Scherer, L.J., Rossi, J.J. Approaches for the sequence-specific knockdown of mRNA. *Nat. Biotechnol.* 2003; 21: 1457–1465.

79. Bertrand, E.L., Rossi, J.J. Facilitation of hammerhead ribozyme catalysis by the nucleocapsid protein of HIV-1 and the heterogeneous nuclear ribonucleoprotein A1. *EMBO J.* 1994; 13: 2904–2912.

80. Bagheri, S., Kashani-Sabet, M. Ribozymes in the age of molecular therapeutics. *Curr. Mol. Med.* 2004; 4: 489–506.

81. Achenbach, J.C., Chiuman, W., Cruz, R.P., Li, Y. DNAzymes: from creation in vitro to application in vivo. *Curr. Pharm. Biotechnol.* 2004; 5: 321–336.

82. Santoro, S.W., Joyce, G.F. A general purpose RNA-cleaving DNA enzyme. *Proc. Natl. Acad. Sci. USA* 1997; 94: 4262–4266.

83. Todd, A.V., Fuery, C.J., Impey, H.L., Applegate, T.L., Haughton, M.A. DzyNA-PCR: use of DNAzymes to detect and quantify nucleic acid sequences in a real-time fluorescent format. *Clin. Chem.* 2000; 46: 625–630.

84. Chen, Y., McMicken, H.W. Intracellular production of DNA enzyme by a novel single-stranded DNA expression vector. *Gene Ther.* 2003; 10: 1776–1780.

85. Gopalan, V., Vioque, A., Altman, S. RNase P: variations and uses. *J. Biol. Chem.* 2002; 277: 6759–6762.

86. Zhu, J., Trang, P., Kim, K., Zhou, T., Deng, H., Liu, F. Effective inhibition of Rta expression and lytic replication of Kaposi's sarcoma-associated herpesvirus by human RNase P. *Proc. Natl. Acad. Sci. USA* 2004; 101: 9073–9078.

87. Yukita, M., Kitano, M., Miyano-Kurosaki, N., Takeuchi, H., Nashimoto, M., Takaku, H. RNA cleavage by a mammalian tRNA 3′-processing endoribonuclease (3′tRNase) reduces HIV-1 expression. *Nucleic Acids Res. Suppl.* 2002; 2: 297–298.

88. Reynolds, A., Leake, D., Boese, Q., Scaringe, S., Marshall, W.S., Khvorova, A. Rational siRNA design for RNA interference. *Nat. Biotechnol.* 2004; 22: 326–330.

89. Wang, L., Mu, F.Y. A Web-based design center for vector-based siRNA and siRNA cassette. *Bioinformatics* 2004; 20: 1818–1820.

90. Jones, S.W., Souza, P.M., Lindsay, M.A. siRNA for Gene silencing: a route to drug target discovery. *Curr. Opin. Pharmacol.* 2004; 4: 522–527.

91. Hemann, M.T., Fridman, J.S., Zilfou, J.T., Hernando, E., Paddison, P.J., Cordon-Cardo, C., Hannon, G.J., Lowe, S.W. An epi-allelic series of p53 hypomorphs created by stable RNAi produces distinct tumor phenotypes in vivo. *Nat. Genet.* 2003; 33: 396–400.

92. Anderson, J., Banerjea, A., Akkina, R. Bispecific short hairpin siRNA constructs targeted to CD4, CXCR4, and CCR5 confer HIV-1 resistance. *Oligonucleotides* 2003; 13: 303–312.

93. Cocks, B.G., Theriault, T.P. Developments in effective application of small inhibitory RNA (siRNA) technology in mammalian cells. *Drug Discovery Today* 2004; 3: 165–171.

94. Matzke, M., Aufsatz, W., Kanno, T., Daxinger, L., Papp, I., Mette, M.F., Matzke, A.J. Genetic analysis of RNA-mediated transcriptional gene silencing. *Biochim. Biophys. Acta* 2004; 1677: 129–141.

95. Wassenegger, M., Heimes, S., Riedel, L., Sanger, H.L. RNA-directed de novo methylation of genomic sequences in plants. *Cell* 1994; 76: 567–576.

96. Morris, K.V., Chan, S.W., Jacobsen, S.E., Looney, D.J. Small interfering RNA-induced transcriptional gene silencing in human cells. *Science* 2004; 305: 1289–1292.

97. Kawasaki, H., Taira, K. Induction of DNA methylation and gene silencing by short interfering RNAs in human cells. *Nature* 2004; 431: 211–217.

98. Powell, S.K., Kaloss, M.A., Pinkstaff, A., McKee, R., Burimski, I., Pensiero, M., Otto, E., Stemmer, W.P., Soong, N.W. Breeding of retroviruses by DNA shuffling for improved stability and processing yields. *Nat. Biotechnol.* 2000; 18: 1279–1282.

99. Tognon, C.E., Kirk, H.E., Passmore, L.A., Whitehead, I.P., Der, C.J., Kay, R.J. Regulation of RasGRP via a phorbol ester-responsive C1 domain. *Mol. Cell Biol.* 1998; 18: 6995–7008.

100. Berquin, I.M., Dziubinski, M.L., Nolan, G.P., Ethier, S.P. A functional screen for genes inducing epidermal growth factor autonomy of human mammary epithelial cells confirms the role of amphiregulin. *Oncogene* 2001; 20: 4019–4028.

101. Douma, S., Van Laar, T., Zevenhoven, J., Meuwissen, R., Van Garderen, E., Peeper, D.S. Suppression of anoikis and induction of metastasis by the neurotrophic receptor TrkB. *Nature* 2004; 430: 1034–1039.

102. Ossovskaya, V.S., Mazo, I.A., Chernov, M.V., Chernova, O.B., Strezoska, Z., Kondratov, R., Stark, G.R., Chumakov, P.M., Gudkov, A.V. Use of genetic suppressor elements to dissect distinct biological effects of separate p53 domains. *Proc. Natl. Acad. Sci. USA* 1996; 93: 10309–10314.

103. Simons, A.H., Dafni, N., Dotan, I., Oron, Y., Canaani, D. Genetic synthetic lethality screen at the single gene level in cultured human cells. *Nucleic Acids Res.* 2001; 29: E100.

104. Novoa, I., Zeng, H., Harding, H.P., Ron, D. Feedback inhibition of the unfolded protein response by GADD34-mediated dephosphorylation of eIF2alpha. *J. Cell Biol.* 2001; 153: 1011–1022.

105. Wunner, W.H., Pallatroni, C., Curtis, P.J. Selection of genetic inhibitors of rabies virus. *Arch. Virol.* 2004; 149: 1653–1662.

106. Neznanov, N., Neznanova, L., Kondratov, R.V., Burdelya, L., Kandel, E.S., O'Rourke, D.M., Ullrich, A., Gudkov, A.V. Dominant negative form of signal-regulatory protein-alpha (SIRPalpha/SHPS-1) inhibits tumor necrosis factor-mediated apoptosis by activation of NF-kappa B. *J. Biol. Chem.* 2003; 278: 3809–3815.

107. Rhoades, K., Wong-Staal, F. Inverse genomics as a powerful tool to identify novel targets for the treatment of neurodegenerative diseases. *Mechanisms Ageing Dev.* 2003; 124: 125–132.

108. Kawasaki, H., Taira, K. A functional gene discovery in the Fas-mediated pathway to apoptosis by analysis of transiently expressed randomized hybrid-ribozyme libraries. *Nucleic Acids Res.* 2002; 30: 3609–3614.

109. Buchholz, C.J., Peng, K.W., Morling, F.J., Zhang, J., Cosset, F.L., Russell, S.J. In vivo selection of protease cleavage sites from retrovirus display libraries. *Nat. Biotechnol.* 1998; 16: 951–954.

110. Aza-Blanc, P., Cooper, C.L., Wagner, K., Batalov, S., Deveraux, Q.L., Cooke, M.P. Identification of modulators of TRAIL-induced apoptosis via RNAi-based phenotypic screening. *Mol. Cell* 2003; 12: 627–637.

111. Silva, J.M., Mizuno, H., Brady, A., Lucito, R., Hannon, G.J. RNA interference microarrays: high-throughput loss-of-function genetics in mammalian cells. *Proc. Natl. Acad. Sci. USA* 2004; 101: 6548–6552.

112. Li, Q.X., Robbins, J.N., Welch, P.J., Wong-Staal, F., Barber, J.R. A novel functional genomics approach identifies mTERT as a suppressor of fibroblast transformation. *Nucleic Acids Res.* 2000; 28: 2605–2612.

7 Use of Protein Microarrays for Molecular Network Analysis and Signal-Pathway Profiling

Katherine R. Calvo, Lance A. Liotta, and Emanuel F. Petricoin

CONTENTS

INTRODUCTION

Human disease is thought to be largely genetic in etiology. Underlying genetic mutations can be inherited through the germ line, or they can occur as the result of somatic mechanisms. Such mutated genes encode altered proteins that perturb normal cellular physiology, resulting in disease. The current ongoing revolution in molecular medicine has begun to elucidate the molecular basis of human disease, with the ultimate goal of developing rationally designed and targeted therapies. This process of investigation has consisted of multiple evolving and overlapping phases. The gene-discovery phase has been largely driven by key technological advances, including polymerase chain reaction (PCR), high-throughput sequencing, and the availability of low-cost computing, all of which have contributed to a revolution in bioinformatics. This phase culminated in the completion of the Human Genome Project in 2003 [1, 2], 50 years following the discovery of the DNA double-helix molecule. Now that the genome-sequencing effort is almost entirely completed, there are ongoing efforts to identify genetic polymorphisms (e.g., single nucleotide polymorphisms [SNPs]) that point to disease predisposition or to unique responses to therapy, such as idiosyncratic drug side effects [3].

Development of gene microarrays brought about the functional genomics phase in which relative expression from thousands of genes can be measured at once, which can be employed to correlate gene-expression patterns with disease classification and predict response to therapy. Gene-expression profiles have been demonstrated as a new approach to molecular taxonomy and can subclassify and predict outcomes for complex entities such as lymphoma [4–6], prostate cancer [7], breast cancer [8], and ovarian cancer [9].

Although DNA is the information archive of the cell, the execution of the disease process occurs through altered protein function. While gene microarray studies elucidate gene-expression patterns associated with disease, they give no indication of the complexity of protein–protein interactions, their localization, or whether the encoded proteins are stably expressed, phosphorylated, cleaved, acetylated, glycosylated, or functionally "active." For many diseases, such as cancer, protein function can be dramatically altered, and key signaling pathways that regulate critical cellular functions, including proliferation, apoptosis, differentiation, survival, immunity, metabolism, invasion, and metastasis, are ultimately affected. The elucidation of which molecular networks are deranged will be critical for the development of effective combinations of pharmacologic inhibitors [10]. Proteomic expression profiling can provide a new opportunity for a systems-biology approach to disease that can synergize with genomic and transcriptomic analysis. The next phase of the molecular-medicine revolution will involve the use of genomic technologies combined with newly evolving proteomic technologies for improved diagnosis and prognosis. This combination will drive the development of individualized molecularly targeted therapies, ushering in a new era of clinical medicine.

HISTORICAL CONTEXT OF
TISSUE-BASED PROFILING

In the past, tissue-based diagnosis of human disease has largely occurred under the rubric of the medical specialty of anatomic pathology. Despite the recent advances in medical science, we still rely on the well-trained human eye of a pathologist for tissue diagnosis and classification. Diagnosis is largely made on the basis of morphology and pattern recognition involving multiple variables, including tissue architecture, cellular configurations, pleomorphism, nuclear shape and contour, and staining patterns. For example, cancer cells typically have higher nuclear-to-cytoplasmic ratios, prominent nucleoli, distinctive chromatin patterns, and a high mitotic index. Accurate diagnosis requires years of experience, as benign reactive conditions can also exhibit similar characteristics. Immunohistochemical analysis and use of antibody stains for subclassification of tumors has recently added a much-improved dimension to tissue-based clinical diagnostics. However, although tumors often display the same histologic and immunohistochemical profiles, there is a wide range of patient response to treatments. This disparity suggests that there is a diverse biology of tumors on a molecular level that is not apparent by outward microscopic morphology. For example, diffuse large B-cell lymphoma has a very heterogeneous outcome pattern. Gene microarray studies have been able uncover several distinct gene-expression patterns that correlate with distinct patient outcome patterns not readily apparent by pathologic analysis [4, 5, 11]. It is likely that the differential gene-expression patterns seen in these examples give rise to unique combinations of protein products that cooperate along multiple deranged signaling pathways and ultimately regulate the malignancy in a patient-specific manner. The complex portrait of functional protein expression is predicted to contain important information about the pathologic process taking place in the cells within their tissue microenvironment. This proteomic information ultimately will contain valuable information for diagnostic classification of tumors, for prognosis, and more importantly, for therapeutic targeting [12].

Once disease has been diagnosed and characterized, the identification of specific derangements within the molecular networks serves as the basis for the formulation of personalized molecularly targeted therapeutic strategies [13]. The ability to characterize information flow through known protein–protein-signaling networks that interconnect the extracellular tissue microenvironment to the intracellular transcriptional regulatory processes will be the nexus for patient-specific therapy. Using cancer as a model, the malignant phenotype is the culmination of multiple genetic or epigenetic "hits" [14, 15], which cooperate to change and modulate protein function along multiple protein-signaling pathways regulating cellular physiologic processes including proliferation, differentiation, apoptosis, metabolism, immune recognition, invasion, and metastasis. Many approaches to elucidating altered protein function in human disease have relied on the use of *in vitro* cultured cell lines originally derived from fresh tissue. However, cultured cells may not accurately represent the molecular events taking place in the actual tissue they were derived from. Protein expression levels and posttranslational modifications affecting protein activity of the cultured cells are influenced by the culture environment, and these properties can be quite different from those of the proteins expressed in the native tissue state. This is because the cultured cells have inevitably lost the contextuality of the *in situ* tissue elements that regulate gene expression, such as soluble factors, extracellular matrix molecules, and cell–cell communication. Human disease occurs in the context of complex tissue microenvironments [16] involving host stromata, immune cells, cytokines, and growth factors that may not be adequately reflected in either *in vitro* studies or nonhuman animal studies. In the context of clinical medicine and patient treatment, individual biologic heterogeneity must be taken into consideration. In fact, it is predictable that each patient can harbor unique attributes that are critical, for example, to an understanding of the tumor–host behavior that can be utilized for effective tailored therapeutic targeting.

PROTEIN-MICROARRAY TECHNOLOGIES
FOR CLINICAL APPLICATIONS

Until recently it was not realistic to perform detailed proteomic analysis of individual patient biopsy specimens due to the relatively large amount of material that was required by "traditional" proteomic technologies, such as two-dimensional polyacrylamide gel electrophoresis analysis or multiplexed Western blotting. Because there is no equivalent protein amplification that compares with PCR-based amplification of DNA, the analysis of low-abundance protein analytes from minute quantities of tissue cells was virtually impossible. However, recent technological developments of highly sensitive, specific, and semiquantitative protein-microarray systems [16, 17] have proven very powerful. These platforms allow the experimentalist to capture the dynamic phosphoprotein-signaling networks in small patient biopsies from as little as 10,000 cells. Pure populations of diseased cells and surrounding host tissue are segregated via laser-capture microdissection (LCM) [18] technologies. LCM allows the procurement and extraction of a microscopic homogeneous cellular subpopulation from its complex tissue milieu under direct microscopic visualization [18–21]. With this technology, a pure subpopulation can be analyzed and compared with adjacent stromal cells, epithelial cells, or any interacting populations of cells within the same tissue. The integrity of cellular proteins is preserved during microdissection, which allows for subsequent quantitative analysis in gene or protein microarrays or MS analysis. The molecular analysis of pathologic processes in clinical specimens can be significantly enhanced by procurement of pure populations of cells from complex tissue biopsies using LCM [22, 23]. The next-generation automated LCM platforms allow the experimentalist to microscopically inspect patient biopsies, identify and highlight distinct cellular populations on a computer monitor, and then automatically collect the selected diseased cells for molecular analysis using robotic processes.

Mapping of cell-signaling networks is achieved by using multiple validated panels of antibodies. For example, our laboratory, with help from the laboratory of Dr. Gordon Mills at M.D. Anderson Cancer Center, has validated several hundred antibodies to date (posted at http://home.ccr.cancer.gov/ncifdaproteomics/) against key regulatory proteins and their posttranslationally modified forms (i.e., phosphorylated, cleaved, acetylated, etc.). In theory, the functional state of up to 100 phosphospecific end points can be assessed from cells contained within a single 1-cm biopsy. The ensuing "wiring diagram" maps reveal the functional state of multiple protein "nodes" along multiple interconnected pathways [19], thereby determining the activity of information flow driving aberrant gene transcription and cell function in the context of disease. In the future, a clinical oncologist could use this information to devise cocktails and combinations of specific inhibitors to pharmacologically target multiple nodes along pathogenic pathways in efforts to shut down aberrant signaling within an individual patient's specific tumor or disease [20]. Importantly, response to therapy could be monitored over time, with appropriate adjustments to the therapy as the tumor recurred (Figure 7.1).

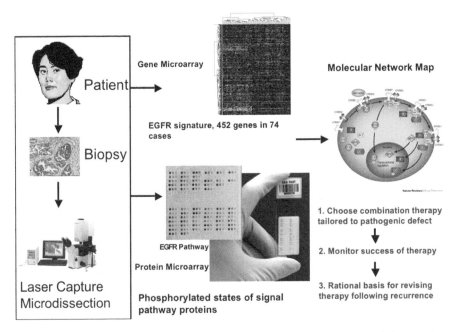

Gene Microarray

Molecular Network Map

Patient

EGFR signature, 452 genes in 74 cases

Biopsy

EGFR Pathway

Protein Microarray

Laser Capture
Microdissection

Phosphorylated states of signal pathway proteins

1. Choose combination therapy tailored to pathogenic defect

2. Monitor success of therapy

3. Rational basis for revising therapy following recurrence

FIGURE 7.1 Implementation of molecular profiling for individualized targeted therapeutics. Following biopsy and laser-capture microdissection, a molecular description of the tumor can be generated using both gene-transcript profiling and protein-microarray signal-pathway analysis. Therapies can then be selected to address specific molecular defects in the tumor. Following initiation of treatment, biopsies can be obtained to determine whether the selected therapy is having the desired biochemical effect as well as determining whether the tumor has upregulated other resistance mechanisms that may require modification of therapy. Should recurrence of the disease occur, the tumor could then be rebiopsied and therapies chosen again in a rational pattern based upon the signaling abnormalities detected.

PROTEIN-MICROARRAY FORMATS

There are two major classes of protein microarrays: forward-phase arrays (FPA) and reverse-phase arrays (RPA) (Figure 7.2). For analysis of clinical patient specimens, we have found RPAs to be inherently superior, with many advantages over the use of FPAs.

When using FPAs, the antibodies, or bait molecules, are adherent to a substratum, such as a nitrocellulose-coated glass slide. The FPA array can, in theory, provide simultaneous information about many analytes from a single lysate, since each spot represents a different immobilized antibody. The FPA array is incubated with one patient's cellular lysate (e.g., cells procured from a tumor), and an attempt is made to measure the expression or activity of multiple proteins on one array. This approach has several obstacles that ultimately need to be overcome for optimal performance.

Forward Phase Protein Microarray

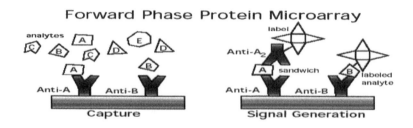

Reverse Phase Protein Microarray

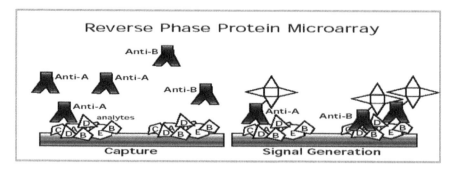

FIGURE 7.2 Classes of protein-microarray technology. Forward-phase arrays (top) immobilize a bait molecule such as an antibody designed to capture specific analytes with a mixture of test sample proteins. The bound analytes are detected by a second sandwich antibody or by labeling the analyte directly (upper right). Reverse-phase arrays (bottom) immobilize the test sample analytes (e.g., lysate from laser-capture microdissected cells) on the solid phase. An analyte-specific ligand (e.g., antibody) is applied in solution phase (lower left). Bound antibodies are detected by secondary tagging and signal amplification (lower right).

Firstly, if a protein of interest is to be detected, it must be captured by the immobilized antibody, which recognizes one epitope. The array is often subsequently incubated with a second labeled antibody for detection, called a "sandwich assay." The second antibody must recognize a different epitope on the same patient's protein. The concentrations of the target protein and the antibody should be optimally matched relative to their affinity constants to identify the relevant linear detection range. Because there are two sets of affinity constants for each patient protein analyzed (corresponding to the immobilized and the second antibody), the use of this format doubles the stringency placed on detection linearity for each spot across the array. In addition, many approaches attempt to amplify the signal of the target proteins by direct conjugation with a fluorescent or biotin tag. Such conjugation often denatures, damages, or masks the epitope recognized by the immobilized antibody, and thus a blank spot on the array may not be reflective of the underlying analyte concentration.

Conversely, with the RPA (Figure 7.2), individual lysates are immobilized on the array. Each array can contain many lysates from different patient samples that are incubated with one antibody. The antibody levels are measured and directly compared across many samples. For this reason, RPAs do not require direct labeling of the patient proteins and do not utilize a two-site antibody sandwich. Hence, there is no experimental variability introduced due to labeling yield, efficiency, or epitope

Reverse Phase Protein Microarray Layout

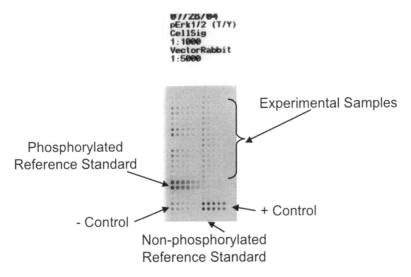

FIGURE 7.3 Typical reverse-phase protein-microarray format. A new type of protein array is the reverse-phase array in which, unlike antibody arrays, the cellular lysate is immobilized on a treated slide (e.g., nitrocellulose). Lysates are prepared from cultured cells or microdissected tissues and then are arrayed in miniature dilution curves (diluted from left to right) such that any given analyte can be evaluated within the linear dynamic ranges of the antibody and analyte affinities and concentrations. The analyte molecule contained in the sample is then detected by a separate labeled probe (e.g., antibody) applied to the surface of the array. This array is highly linear, very sensitive, and requires no labeling of the sample proteins. A reference standard consisting of a cocktail of phosphorylated peptides is used as an invariant control and placed on each array. A positive and negative control lysate is also arrayed as a control for the phosphospecific antibodies.

masking. Each array comprises dozens of patient samples, allowing subtle differences in a target protein to be measured, as each sample is exposed for the same amount of time to the same concentrations of primary and secondary antibody and amplification reagents. Additionally, each lysate can be applied as a miniature dilution curve on the RPA array, along with reference standards and positive and negative controls (Figure 7.3) [21]. This provides an excellent means of (a) matching the antibody concentration with the target protein concentration so that the linear range of detection is ensured to exist on at least one or more diluted spots and (b) converting the relative intensity values obtained to an invariant reference standard unit. The high sensitivity of RPAs is partly explained by the fact that the antibody can be tagged and the signal amplified independent of the immobilized patient sample. For example, coupling the detection antibody with highly sensitive tyramide-based avidin/biotin signal-amplification systems can yield detection sensitivities down to fewer than 1000 to 5000 molecules/spot. A biopsy of 50,000 cells can yield over 50 RPA arrays, with each array being probed by a different antibody. RPAs have been successfully applied to analyze the state of mediators of apoptosis [21, 22] and mitogenesis pathways within microdissected premalignant lesions, and the results can be compared with adjacent normal epithelium, invasive carcinoma, and host stroma [23, 24]. RPAs are particularly well suited to the mapping of signal-transduction pathways in cancer cell lines [25] and patient specimens [19, 21–24, 26].

MAPPING MOLECULAR NETWORK ANALYSIS FROM CLINICAL SPECIMENS

Proteins are assembled into complex networks through a variety of protein–protein interactions in both extracellular and intracellular microenvironments. The structural conformation of a protein and the subsequent access of interaction domains (e.g., SH2 and SH3 domains) enable a highly selective recognition between protein partners in a communication circuit of protein–protein interactions. Proteins can undergo conformational changes that functionally permit or prevent protein activity within networks. Conformational changes are largely dictated by posttranslational modifications that include phosphorylation, cleavage, acetylation, glycosylation, and ubiquitinylation. Such modifications functionally define regulated protein–protein interactions through specific domain binding, which then controls the information flow from the extracellular space to the nucleus. These signaling networks regulate key biologic processes defining cell function within larger tissue- and organ-specific contexts. In cancer, specific protein-signaling networks are typically deranged, resulting in unregulated proliferation, aberrant differentiation, and immortality, which ultimately underpins the malignant process. Aberrant activity through specific signaling pathways can be monitored by evaluating the phosphorylation of proteins within key nodes as a multiplexed kinase substrate assay. This can be achieved by using antibodies that recognize the active form (e.g., phosphorylated) of a protein versus the inactive form (e.g., unphosphorylated). Disruption of key regulated protein–protein interactions in diseased cells very often serves as an important indicator of drug-therapy targets [10].

Coupled with LCM, RPAs offer the advantage of allowing (a) the evaluation of native proteins in normal and diseased cells and (b) the posttranslational modifications associated with protein–protein interactions [16, 21], under the assumption that information flow through a specific "node" in the proteomic network requires the phosphorylation of a known protein at a specific amino acid sequence. By measuring the proportion of those protein molecules that are phosphorylated, we can infer the level of activity of the upstream kinase at that node. For example, we can infer MEK kinase activity by measuring phosphorylation of ERK. If we compare this measurement over time, or at stages of disease progression, or before and after treatment, a correlation can be made between the activity of the kinase and the biologic or disease state. The development of highly sensitive protein microarrays now makes it possible to profile the states of dozens of kinase substrates at once and to provide information about entire protein-signal pathways in tissue biopsies, aspirates, or body fluid samples.

The application of this technology to clinical molecular diagnostics is greatly enhanced by increasing the number of high-quality antibodies that are specific for the modification or activation state of target proteins within key pathways. Antibody specificity is particularly critical given the complex array of biological proteins at the vastly different concentrations contained within cell lysates. Given that there are no standard PCR-like direct amplification methods for proteins, the sensitivity of antibodies must be achieved in the near-femtomolar range. Moreover, the labeling and amplification method must be linear and reproducible. A cubic centimeter of biopsy tissue contains approximately 10^9 cells; in contrast, a needle biopsy or cell aspirate contains fewer than 100,000 cells. If the cell population of the specimen is heterogeneous, the final number of actual tumor cells microdissected or procured for analysis can be as low as a few thousand. Assuming that the proteins of interest, and their phosphorylated counterparts, exist in low abundance, the total concentration of analyte proteins in the sample will be very low. Newer generations of protein microarrays, combined with highly sensitive and specific validated antibodies, are now able to achieve adequate levels of sensitivity for analysis of clinical specimens.

BIOINFORMATIC ANALYSIS OF PROTEIN-MICROARRAY DATA

A variety of methods have been used to analyze data obtained from protein microarrays [22, 25, 27–31]. These methods have been primarily adopted from those used in gene microarray analysis. The analysis of RPAs presents a new set of challenges compared with conventional spotted arrays. Multiple RPAs, each analyzing a different phosphorylated protein, are scanned; the background is subtracted; spot intensities are calculated and normalized; and the dilution curve is collapsed to a single intensity value measured within the linear dynamic range of the reference standard. This value is then assigned a relative normalized intensity value referenced to the other patient samples on the array. The data output is in a form suitable for analysis by traditional unsupervised and supervised bioinformatics computer systems. Ultimately, protein array data are displayed as traditional "heat maps," which can be analyzed by Bayesian clustering methods for signal-pathway profiling (Figure 7.4).

PERSONALIZED MOLECULAR MEDICINE USING PROTEIN-MICROARRAY TECHNOLOGY

Cancer progression is characterized by the accumulation of multiple genetic mutations or epigenetic events that cooperate to drive malignancy. The orchestration of these genetic events occurs via dysregulated communication within signaling pathways that together drive proliferation, promote metastasis, block differentiation, or inhibit apoptosis, thereby conferring "immortality" (Figure 7.5). Each of these cellular processes is regulated by complex protein networks with multiple interconnected nodes of activity. Theoretically, aberrant protein function at any key region within the signaling network can impact the flow of downstream information. In cancer, there could be numerous combinations of "mutated" or aberrant regulatory proteins in different cooperating and interdependent pathways that together are sufficient to drive malignancy. Likewise, each individual patient's cancer might have a unique complement of pathogenic molecular derangements. It is also possible that

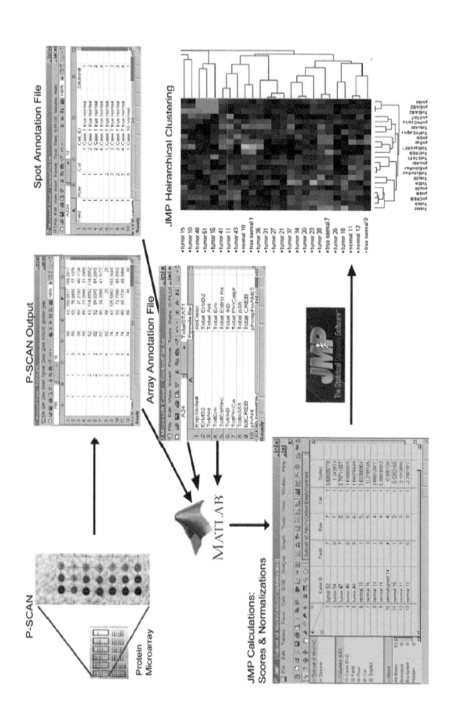

each metastasis residing in different host organ locations can have a unique protein-signaling circuitry that is in part dictated by the specific organ tissue microenvironment. Changes in signaling circuitry as cells undergo metastasis to a distant site has been observed and reported in studies where matched primary ovarian cancer vs. peritoneal metastasis studies were analyzed [22]. We have also found that individual patients who share the same type of cancer, with identical histologic diagnoses, have tumors that display unique *in vivo* proteomic signaling profiles with measurable signaling responses to perfused chemotherapy during surgery [26]. Consequently, a given class of therapy might be effective for only a subset of patients who harbor tumors with susceptible molecular derangements.

In a recent study [32], the activity of signaling networks within specimens obtained from patients with acute myeloid leukemia was evaluated in response to stimulation with cytokines. The investigators noted distinct patterns within phosphoprotein-signaling networks in stimulated leukemic cells that produced patient classifications predictive of outcome. Measuring the responses of protein-signaling pathways in cells obtained from solid tumors to stimuli can also provide useful therapeutic information. Different combinations of functional or redundant pathways can also be revealed upon stimulation. There is a strong justification to develop diagnostic and treatment strategies that would allow a clinical team to formulate a unique combination of molecular inhibitors that would target specific aberrant protein circuits in an individual patient's tumor.

Protein kinases and phosphatases are key regulatory proteins that play a role in controlling information flow between nodes in the cellular signaling circuitry that ultimately regulates gene transcription. Their aberrant function is frequently central to the pathogenesis of cancer and other diseases [33]. C-Src may be a cooperative partner with multiple other oncoproteins in aberrantly remodeling signaling pathways in cancer [34, 35]. Constitutive activation of Ras has been associated with uncontrolled tumor growth in many cancers, including pancreatic, colon, and lung [36]. In addition, Ras can drive expression of IL-8, thereby eliciting a stromal response that fosters angiogenesis and tumor progression [37]. Farnesylation of Ras is one of the key posttranslational modifications required for activity. Hence the use of effective farnesyl transferase inhibitors may be an important component of combinatorial therapies [37].

Until recently, the concept of using molecularly targeted therapies has focused on the development and use of single-agent inhibitors [37–46]. Imatinib (Gleevec, STI-571) is a prime example of the promise that molecularly targeted inhibitors hold as potentially curative therapies [42, 43]. Chronic myelogenous leukemia (CML) is a consequence of the (9;22) chromosomal translocation that encodes the chimeric oncoprotein Bcr-Abl, which drives unchecked proliferation of leukemia cells, largely by altering protein-signaling circuits via the constitutively active Abl tyrosine kinase

---

FIGURE 7.4 *(see facing page)* Bioinformatic analysis of multiplexed reverse-phase arrays. Relative, normalized, and background-subtracted intensity values are obtained through the analysis of scanned images of each stained slide. Each analyte is assessed within the linear dynamic range of the reference standard calibrant. The relative intensities are then scaled and analyzed with unsupervised classification programs to generate an unbiased clustering portrait for patients and pathway end points simultaneously.

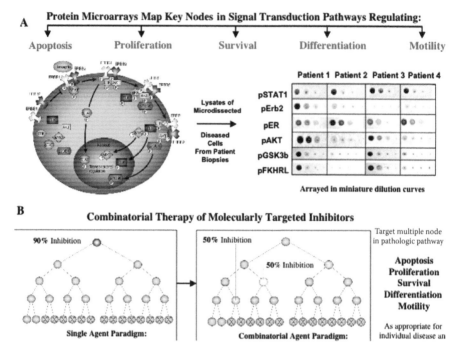

A   Protein Microarrays Map Key Nodes in Signal Transduction Pathways Regulating:

Apoptosis   Proliferation   Survival   Differentiation   Motility

	Patient 1	Patient 2	Patient 3	Patient 4
pSTAT1				
pErb2				
pER				
pAKT				
pGSK3b				
pFKHRL				

Lysates of Microdissected

→

Diseased Cells From Patient Biopsies

Arrayed in miniature dilution curves

B   Combinatorial Therapy of Molecularly Targeted Inhibitors

90% Inhibition

50% Inhibition

50% Inhibition

Target multiple node in pathologic pathway

**Apoptosis
Proliferation
Survival
Differentiation
Motility**

As appropriate for individual disease an

Single Agent Paradigm: **Combinatorial Agent Paradigm:**

FIGURE 7.5 Functional proteomic profiling of human disease for individualized combina-torial therapy. (A) Protein microarrays map the functional state of key nodes in signal-transduction pathways orchestrating human disease. Protein-signaling pathways consist of complex networks of regulatory proteins that become activated via posttranslational modifi-cations (e.g., phosphorylation) through protein–protein interactions. Microarrays containing pure populations of diseased cells (e.g., tumor cells) are assayed for the phosphorylated form of key phosphoproteins using phosphospecific antibodies. Activity of up to 50–100 signaling nodes can be assayed from a single patient biopsy. These data are used to create a signaling circuitry map of the diseased cells identifying pathologic pathways suitable for targeting with pharmacologic inhibitors. (B) Combinatorial therapy as a model for treatment of disease using molecularly targeted inhibitors. Traditional pharmacologic inhibitors have been used to inhibit one key activated regulator within a signal-transduction cascade in efforts to effectively shut down up to 90% of the pathway using a high dose of the agent. In a combinatorial therapy model, the same level of inhibition can be achieved using inhibitors to multiple nodes along the pathway using lower doses of pharmacologic inhibitors.

portion of the protein. Treatment with imatinib targets the Abl protein kinase by binding to and blocking its ATP-binding domain. Imatinib has a striking ability to induce remission in CML patients, even when their leukemia is resistant to traditional chemotherapy. A key advantage of molecularly targeted agents like imatinib is their specificity and lack of host toxicity as compared with classical chemotherapy or radiation treatments. Imatinib can also target c-kit (stem cell factor receptor) and platelet-derived growth-factor receptor (PDGFR). Hence, it has shown some utility for the treatment of gastrointestinal stromal tumors (GIST) and dermatofibrosarcoma protuberans (DFSP).

CONCLUDING REMARKS AND A VIEW
TO THE FUTURE

A therapeutic regime in the future will likely be one in which a cocktail of selected inhibitors, chosen based on the patient-specific molecular network (Figure 7.5), are applied concomitantly. Theoretically, if multiple agents along a pathway are used together to mitigate aberrant signaling, lower effective doses of each inhibitor within the cocktail could be used than if one agent were used alone to inhibit the same pathway [10, 47, 48]. Because drug toxicities are largely dose dependent, the use of multiple inhibitors may achieve a higher efficacy with lower toxicity or decreased side effects [10, 47, 48]. The concept of using combinatorial inhibitor therapy has been explored, for example with the epidermal growth-factor receptor (EGFR) tyrosine kinase inhibitor ZD1839 (Iressa) and the anti-Erb-B2 monoclonal antibody trastuzumab (Herceptin) [49]. *In vitro* studies show synergistic inhibition of tumor growth with combined therapy. Thus, the ultimate goal of molecular profiling is not only to provide prognostic information (i.e., responders vs. nonresponders), but to map deranged pathway activation to define the optimal set of interconnected drug targets.

Drug-discovery efforts are intensely focused on the development of additional kinase inhibitors [42]. The effective development of a cadre of specific and selective inhibitors will be necessary components in the expansion of combinatorial individualized therapies. Despite the initial success of molecularly targeted therapeutics for certain cancers, such as imatinib, many patients relapse with resistant tumor cells after a period of remission. The development of resistance to single-agent therapy underscores the need to combine multiple agents, which would theoretically be more effective than single agents alone. In addition to kinase inhibitors, other classes of molecules may also prove to be useful targets, such as (a) caspases, which are modified by cleavage and are involved in apoptosis, or (b) histone acetylases and deacetylases, which regulate gene transcription. At present, multiple molecules that block kinase activity are being investigated in phase III trials, and as many as 30 kinase inhibitors are being evaluated in phase I/II trials [44–46]. The simultaneous development of enabling data-generating technologies, such as protein-microarray platforms, is a necessary component to effective and strategic targeted medicine. The ability of clinical investigators to develop a portrait of the molecular network of a diseased cell — and then, armed with this information, to choose and select combinations of targeted therapeutics — could herald the next revolution in molecular medicine.

DISCLAIMER

The views expressed here are expressed solely by the authors and should not be construed as representative of those of the Department of Health and Human Services, the U.S. Food and Drug Administration. Moreover, aspects of the topics discussed have been filed as U.S. government-owned patent applications. Drs. Petricoin and Liotta are coinventors on these applications and may receive royalties provided under U.S. law.

REFERENCES

1. Lander, E.S., et al., Initial sequencing and analysis of the human genome. *Nature*, 2001. 409 (6822): 860–921.
2. Venter, J.C., et al.
3. Badano, J.L., and Katsanis, N., Beyond Mendel: an evolving view of human genetic disease transmission. *Nat. Rev. Genet.*, 2002. 3 (10): 779–89.
4. Staudt, L.M., Gene expression profiling of lymphoid malignancies. *Annu. Rev. Med.*, 2002. 53: 303–18.
5. Shipp, M.A., et al., Diffuse large B-cell lymphoma outcome prediction by gene-expression profiling and supervised machine learning. *Nat. Med.*, 2002. 8 (1): 68–74.
6. Dave, S.S., et al., Prediction of survival in follicular lymphoma based on molecular features of tumor-infiltrating immune cells. *N. Engl. J. Med.*, 2004. 351 (21): 2159–69.
7. Singh, D., et al., Gene expression correlates of clinical prostate cancer behavior. *Cancer Cell*, 2002. 1 (2): 203–9.
8. Sorlie, T., et al., Repeated observation of breast tumor subtypes in independent gene expression data sets. *Proc. Natl. Acad. Sci. USA*, 2003. 100 (14): 8418–23.
9. Schwartz, D.R., et al., Gene expression in ovarian cancer reflects both morphology and biological behavior, distinguishing clear cell from other poor-prognosis ovarian carcinomas. *Cancer Res.*, 2002. 62 (16): 4722–9.
10. Petricoin, E.F., et al., Clinical proteomics: translating benchside promise into bedside reality. *Nat. Rev. Drug Discov.*, 2002. 1 (9): 683–95.
11. Calvo, K.R., et al., Molecular profiling provides evidence of primary mediastinal large B-cell lymphoma as a distinct entity related to classic Hodgkin lymphoma: implications for mediastinal gray zone lymphomas as an intermediate form of B-cell lymphoma. *Adv. Anat. Pathol.*, 2004. 11 (5): 227–38.
12. Petricoin, E.F., and Liotta, L.A., Clinical applications of proteomics. *J. Nutr.*, 2003. 133 (7, Suppl.): 2476S–84S.
13. Liotta, L.A., Kohn, E.C., and Petricoin, E.F., Clinical proteomics: personalized molecular medicine. *JAMA*, 2001. 286 (18): 2211–4.
14. Moolgavkar, S.H., and Knudson, A.G., Jr., Mutation and cancer: a model for human carcinogenesis. *J. Natl. Cancer Inst.*, 1981. 66 (6): 1037–52.
15. Hanahan, D., and Weinberg, R.A., The hallmarks of cancer. *Cell*, 2000. 100 (1): 57–70.
16. Liotta, L.A., et al., Protein microarrays: meeting analytical challenges for clinical applications. *Cancer Cell*, 2003. 3 (4): 317–25.
17. Espina, V., et al., Use of proteomic analysis to monitor responses to biological therapies. *Expert Opin. Biol. Ther.*, 2004. 4 (1): 83–93.
18. Emmert-Buck, M.R., et al., Laser capture microdissection. *Science*, 1996. 274 (5289): 998–1001.
19. Petricoin, E.F., et al., Mapping molecular networks using proteomics: a vision for patient-tailored combination therapy, 2004 (in submission).
20. Petricoin, E., et al., Clinical proteomics: revolutionizing disease detection and patient tailoring therapy. *J. Proteome Res.*, 2004. 3 (2): 209–17.
21. Paweletz, C.P., et al., Reverse phase protein microarrays which capture disease progression show activation of pro-survival pathways at the cancer invasion front. *Oncogene*, 2001. 20 (16): 1981–9.
22. Sheehan, K.M., et al., Use of reverse phase protein microarrays and reference standard development for molecular network analysis of metastatic ovarian carcinoma. *Mol. Cell Proteomics*, 2005. 4 (4): 346–55.

23. Grubb, R.L., et al., Signal pathway profiling of prostate cancer using reverse phase protein arrays. *Proteomics*, 2003. 3 (11): 2142–6.

24. Wulfkuhle, J.D., et al., Signal pathway profiling of ovarian cancer from human tissue specimens using reverse-phase protein microarrays. *Proteomics*, 2003. 3 (11): 2085–90.

25. Nishizuka, S., et al., Proteomic profiling of the NCI-60 cancer cell lines using new high-density reverse-phase lysate microarrays. *Proc. Natl. Acad. Sci. USA*, 2003. 100 (24): 14229–34.

26. Calvo, K.R., et al., Clinical proteomics: in vivo molecular signaling profiles of human tumors, pre- and post-tumor perfusion with experimental chemotherapy, 2004 (in preparation).

27. Brazma, A., et al., Minimum information about a microarray experiment (MIAME): toward standards for microarray data. *Nat. Genet.*, 2001. 29 (4): 365–71.

28. Carlisle, A.J., et al., Development of a prostate cDNA microarray and statistical gene expression analysis package. *Mol. Carcinog.*, 2000. 28 (1): 12–22.

29. Cutler, P., Protein arrays: the current state-of-the-art. *Proteomics*, 2003. 3 (1): 3–18.

30. Sreekumar, A., et al., Profiling of cancer cells using protein microarrays: discovery of novel radiation-regulated proteins. *Cancer Res.*, 2001. 61 (20): 7585–93.

31. Miller, J.C., et al., Antibody microarray profiling of human prostate cancer sera: antibody screening and identification of potential biomarkers. *Proteomics*, 2003. 3 (1): 56–63.

32. Irish, J.M., et al., Single cell profiling of potentiated phospho-protein networks in cancer cells. *Cell*, 2004. 118 (2): 217–28.

33 Blume-Jensen, P., and Hunter, T., Oncogenic kinase signalling. *Nature*, 2001. 411 (6835): 355–65.

34. Ishizawar, R., and Parsons, S.J., c-Src and cooperating partners in human cancer. *Cancer Cell*, 2004. 6 (3): 209–14.

35. Kloth, M.T., et al., STAT5b, a mediator of synergism between c-Src and the epidermal growth factor receptor. *J. Biol. Chem.*, 2003. 278 (3): 1671–9.

36. Bos, J.L., ras Oncogenes in human cancer: a review. *Cancer Res.*, 1989. 49 (17): 4682–9.

37. Sparmann, A., and Bar-Sagi, D., Ras-induced interleukin-8 expression plays a critical role in tumor growth and angiogenesis. *Cancer Cell*, 2004. 6 (5): 447–58.

38. Crul, M., et al., Ras biochemistry and farnesyl transferase inhibitors: a literature survey. *Anticancer Drugs*, 2001. 12 (3): 163–84.

39. Jones, A.L., and Leyland-Jones, B., Optimizing treatment of HER2-positive metastatic breast cancer. *Semin. Oncol.*, 2004. 31 (5, Suppl. 10): 29–34.

40. Leyland-Jones, B., Trastuzumab: hopes and realities. *Lancet Oncol.*, 2002. 3 (3): 137–44.

41. Sebolt-Leopold, J.S., MEK inhibitors: a therapeutic approach to targeting the Ras-MAP kinase pathway in tumors. *Curr. Pharm. Des.*, 2004. 10 (16): 1907–14.

42. Traxler, P., Tyrosine kinases as targets in cancer therapy — successes and failures. *Expert Opin. Ther. Targets*, 2003. 7 (2): 215–34.

43. Druker, B.J., Imatinib as a paradigm of targeted therapies. *Adv. Cancer Res.*, 2004. 91: 1–30.

44. Tibes, R., Trent, J., and Kurzrock, R., Tyrosine kinase inhibitors and the dawn of molecular cancer therapeutics. *Annu. Rev. Pharmacol. Toxicol.*, 2005. 45:357–84.

45. Traxler, P., et al., Tyrosine kinase inhibitors: from rational design to clinical trials. *Med. Res. Rev.*, 2001. 21 (6): 499–512.

46. Zwick, E., Bange, J., and Ullrich, A., Receptor tyrosine kinases as targets for anticancer drugs. *Trends Mol. Med.*, 2002. 8 (1): 17–23.

47. Araujo, R.P., Doran, C., Liotta, L.A., and Petricoin, E.F., Network-targeted combination therapy: a new concept in cancer treatment. *Drug Discov. Today*, 2005. 1 (4): 425–33.

48. Araujo, R.P., Petricoin, E.F., and Liotta, L.A., A mathematical model of combination therapy using the EGFR signaling network. *Biosystems*, 2005. 80 (1): 57–69.

49. Normanno, N., et al., Cooperative inhibitory effect of ZD1839 (Iressa) in combination with trastuzumab (Herceptin) on human breast cancer cell growth. *Ann. Oncol.*, 2002. 13 (1): 65–72.

8 Laser-Microdissection-Based Transcriptomics Using Microarrays

*Fredrik Kamme, Bernd Meurers, Jessica Zhu,
Da-Thao Tran, Jingxue Yu, Changlu Liu,
Andrew Carmen, and Bingren Hu*

CONTENTS

INTRODUCTION

Laser microdissection is a microscope-based method to isolate one, or many, cells of interest from a tissue section. Two independent technical solutions were developed in 1996–1997 (Emmert-Buck et al., 1996; Bohm et al., 1997). Just before that, in 1995, microarrays had been developed (Lipshutz et al., 1995; Schena et al., 1995). The timing was fortuitous, as laser microdissection provided a means of making microarray analysis specific in complex tissues, and microarray analyses early became a major application for laser microdissection. The list of laser-microdissection applications has grown since then, and it now encompasses transcriptomics (Luo et al., 1999), genomics (Rook et al., 2004), and proteomics (Ornstein et al., 2000; Ahram et al., 2002). This review focuses on the application of laser microdissection in transcriptomics. There are a variety of methods to profile the expression of genes in cells. Among the techniques that globally measure gene expression, microarrays are predominant. Microarrays have technical properties that need to be considered in conjunction with the RNA amplification and labeling systems used to generate a labeled hybridization target. We will thus focus on microarray-based transcriptomics as combined with laser microdissection.

LASER MICRODISSECTION AND RNA QUALITY

Two principles account for all laser microdissection: (a) attaching cells to a cap by localized laser-mediated activation of the cap surface and then lifting the cap off the tissue section (Molecular Devices, Sunnyvale, CA) or (b) freeing cells from the surrounding tissue using a cutting laser and then collecting the isolated cells (Molecular Machines & Industries, Glattbrugg, Switzerland; Leica, Bannockburn, IL; PALM Microlaser Technologies, Bernried, Germany; Zeiss, Thornwood, NY). A recently developed system combines both principles (Veritas™, Molecular Devices). We have experience from both cutting- and attachment-based cell collection of single cells up to hundreds of cells and have found utility in both approaches. An issue of concern is the quality of RNA in the cells collected, due to deleterious effects during tissue fixation (Goldsworthy et al., 1999), during the staining procedure (Burgemeister et al., 2003), or during the laser microdissection itself. Such concerns are clearly warranted, as endogenous RNAses might be active during the staining procedure, and spillover UV laser light used during cutting might damage RNA in adjacent cells.

We have compared RNA from air-dried rat brain sections with that from cresyl-violet-stained sections by quantitative reverse-transcriptase–polymerase chain reaction (RT-PCR) for a specific gene and found no difference (Figure 8.1). PCR measures cDNA, which is really the species of interest, as RNA amplification proceeds via a cDNA intermediate. On the other hand, we have also found that, in the rat gut,

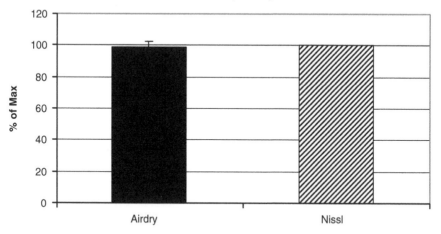

FIGURE 8.1 Quantitative RT-PCR measurement of neuron-specific enolase (NSE) cDNA from tissue sections. Total RNA was extracted from tissue sections that were either air dried directly on the slide or were fixed in acetone and stained using cresyl violet as described by Kamme et al. (2003). RNA was reverse transcribed and cDNA was quantified using quantitative PCR using SYBR green detection on a Smartcycler as described by Kamme et al. (2003). No loss of RNA could be detected during cresyl-violet staining. Two tissue sections per treatment. Error bars indicate standard deviation. Error bar for Nissl group too small to be visible.

even a brief period (30 s) in aqueous media severely depletes RNA (data not shown), probably due to endogenous RNAse activity. Clearly, RNA preservation during tissue staining has to be evaluated for every tissue. We have successfully analyzed gene expression in single dorsal root ganglion neurons using the PALM instrument (Zhu et al., 2004), with the results arguing against gross destruction of RNA in adjacent tissue due to spillover of laser light.

A quality measure of the whole assembled system, which includes RNA quality, RNA amplification, and array analysis, is to assess reproducibility of replicate laser-microdissected samples. We compared 7 samples of 100 rat hippocampal CA1 cells, each collected using PixCell II (Molecular Devices), amplified using the TargetAmp kit (Epicentre Technologies, Madison, WI), and analyzed using cDNA arrays (Figure 8.2). Even though the experiment was done to test the reproducibility of the amplification system, the high reproducibility (average $\log_2 R = .99$) is indicative of good RNA quality. It could be argued that the RNA quality of a single laser-microdissected cell is still a matter of contention, but we believe that this will be more an issue of the properties of the RNA amplification system, which brings us to the matter of sufficiently amplifying the minute amounts of RNA extracted from the laser-microdissected cells.

RNA AMPLIFICATION

RNA amplification is needed to generate the 0.5–10 µg of RNA needed for a typical microarray analysis, starting from the approximately 10–100-pg total RNA/cell that is recovered from a laser-microdissected sample. This is technically challenging, as attested by the multitude of papers on T7 RNA polymerase-based RNA amplification (Phillips and Eberwine, 1996; Pabon et al., 2001; Zhao et al., 2002; Gomes et al., 2003; Li et al., 2003; Polacek et al., 2003; Spiess et al., 2003; Xiang et al., 2003; Goff et al., 2004; Ji et al., 2004; Kamme et al., 2004; Moll et al., 2004; Rudnicki et al., 2004; Schneider et al., 2004). T7 RNA polymerase-based and PCR-based techniques were developed in 1990 (Brady et al., 1990; Van Gelder et al., 1990) and have evolved into several different versions following attempts to improve amplification yield and throughput. More recently, NuGEN's isothermal amplification system added a new amplification principle. There are several commercial kits of the T7 system available today from a variety of vendors, including Affymetrix, Agilent, Ambion, Molecular Devices, Artus-Biotech, Enzo Life Science, Epicentre Technologies, Genisphere, Roche, Stratagene, and System Biosciences. For laser-microdissected samples, a two-round system is normally required.

Considering the sensitivity of RNA amplification to variations in reagent quality, it is probably advisable to at least start off with a commercial kit. Might one avoid RNA amplification issues by simple gross dissection of the tissue and a microarray screen with subsequent confirmation of interesting genes by *in situ* hybridization? Not really, and the explanation reveals one of the limitations of microarrays. While a typical microarray may have a sensitivity of approximately 1/200,000 to 1/500,000, the complexity of a single cell may be 500,000 individual transcripts or higher. Therefore, if a sample is even moderately complex in terms of cell types, there will certainly be a

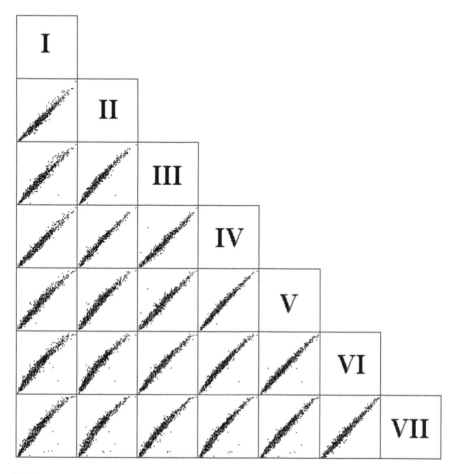

FIGURE 8.2 Pairwise scatter plots of seven laser-microdissected samples from rat hippocampus CA1. Approximately 100 cells were captured per sample using PixCell2 (Molecular Devices). Extracted RNA was amplified using TargetAmp (Epicentre Technologies) and hybridized to cDNA arrays as described by Kamme et al. (2003). Plots show $\log_2$-transformed, quantile-normalized intensity data. Samples are indicated by Roman numerals I–VII. The overall average Pearson's correlation (R^2) was .97.

substantial number of expressed genes that fall below the detection limit and become false negatives. In essence, the microarray has a limited bandwidth. To illustrate this point, we used microarrays to analyze the expression of tyrosine hydroxylase in microdissected *substantia nigra* and in total rat brain RNA. Tyrosine hydroxylase is highly expressed in the *substantia nigra* and gave a high signal-to-noise ratio in the microdissected sample. However, in the whole-brain sample, it was not detectable (Table 8.1), clearly showing the negative effect of increased sample complexity. This effect of sample complexity on microarray data is frequently overlooked when assessing RNA amplification methods. A popular measure of RNA amplification

---

TABLE 8.1
Signal-to-Background Ratios for Tyrosine Hydroxylase Expression Using Total Rat Brain RNA or Microdissected *Substantia Nigra*

Sample	Signal/Background
Whole rat brain RNA	1
Microdissected substantia nigra	16

Note: Microdissection was done using PixCell2, and microarray analysis was performed as described by Kamme et al. (2003).

---

quality is to plot the correlation between unamplified and amplified RNA as an indication of linearity, or maintained representation, of amplification. However, the unamplified data most likely omit a large amount of false negatives and, as such, are in fact biased against rare genes. If the amplification procedure increases the number of detectable genes, one might argue that this is a more informative representation of the sample, even if it is at the expense of a poorer correlation with an unamplified sample. Indeed, it has been reported that RNA amplification improves the sensitivity of microarray analysis as compared with using total RNA (Feldman et al., 2002), likely by reducing the complexity of the RNA mix, as nonpolyadenylated RNAs are not efficiently amplified. An analogy would be proteomic analyses, where albumin and other abundant proteins are regularly removed from samples to permit the detection of less abundant proteins by freeing up "bandwidth" of the assay (Georgiou et al., 2001).

ANALYSIS OF ARRAY DATA

The cardinal argument for laser-microdissection-based expression profiling is, however, not technical, but analytical. Laser microdissection allows the user to generate expression data in a defined cellular context. More often than not, the significance of expression of a particular gene depends on the identity of the cell harboring it. Perhaps the biggest challenge in microarray experiments lies in the analysis of the data generated. Gene-by-gene analysis is time consuming, relies on presumed functions of genes, and cannot capture complex phenomena. Examples of going beyond gene-by-gene analysis are mapping of expression data onto pathways, such as those provided by Ingenuity™ (Mountain View, CA) and Jubilant Biosys (Columbia, MD), pattern matching (Hughes et al., 2000), and network analyses (Tavazoie et al., 1999; Wille et al., 2004). A discussion of microarray data analysis is beyond the scope of this chapter, and the reader is referred to several recent reviews (Sherlock, 2001; de la Fuente et al., 2002; Kaminski and Friedman, 2002; Hariharan, 2003; Leung and Cavalieri, 2003).

Some of the more advanced types of analyses use expression data as a snapshot of the cell "system." To ensure that this snapshot represents a particular state of the cell system, the cell sample must be homogeneous. Accordingly, much of the pattern-matching and network-modeling analyses has been performed on cell culture, or yeast, data. The application of these analysis tools to expression data from *in vivo* models is needed, and laser microdissection will be required to provide the necessary cell-sample homogeneity from many tissues. Sample homogeneity also clearly increases the possibility of seeing coordinate regulation of genes within a given pathway. This opens new statistical possibilities. When several genes within an a priori defined pathway are tested, the statistical probability that the pathway is regulated is a function of all the parts of the pathway. Thus, several genes that are modestly, and statistically insignificantly, regulated may together show that a shared pathway is significantly regulated (Mootha et al., 2003). Due to the large number of data points, microarrays may actually be more sensitive than quantitative PCR of a smaller number of genes for detecting pathway regulation in such a fashion.

APPLICATIONS

Most of the biological applications of expression profiling using laser microdissection and microarrays deal with identifying markers for cell types (Luo et al., 1999; Bonaventure et al., 2002; Kamme et al., 2003; Burbach et al., 2004; Mutsuga et al., 2004; Torres-Munoz et al., 2004), for disease (Peterson et al., 2004), or for tumors (Ma et al., 2003; Nishidate et al., 2004). These are probably the easiest applications from an analytical point of view, as marker genes need not be discussed with regard to their function. Application of laser-microdissection-based expression profiling to characterize disease processes in the central nervous system (CNS) is under way in our laboratory and in others as well. Apart from the more demanding analysis of such data, it has also become clear that sample throughput requirements increase significantly. This is in part due to the fact that gene-expression changes in disease can be highly dynamic (Figure 8.3). Capturing the dynamics of changes in disease-caused transcriptomes facilitates analysis of the data, but it also inflates the number of microarrays required. A new challenge for laser-microdissection–RNA-amplification–microarray technologies is to make processing of larger sample numbers practical and affordable. Developments toward higher sample throughput in laser-microdissection instrumentation include PALM's introduction of a 96-well collection system for their laser-microdissection instrument as well as Affymetrix's 96-well ArrayPlate™ and Illumina's Sentrix™ bead arrays for parallelization of microarray formats. We note, however, that no high-throughput version of an RNA amplification method is yet suitable for laser-microdissected samples.

The combination of laser microdissection and microarrays is still young. Since its inception in 1999, the rate of technical development has accelerated on all fronts, especially in the field of RNA amplification. We expect that the improved reliability and throughput of the entire chain of methods will soon be reflected in more-challenging laser-microdissection applications, such as expression profiling of disease processes. We predict that, as techniques for high-throughput RNA amplification are developed, these applications will permit the integration of higher-throughput laser

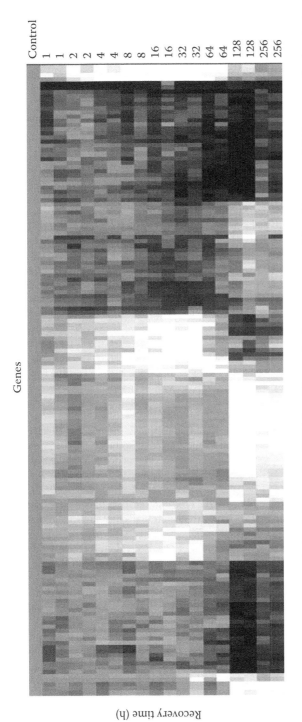

FIGURE 8.3 Dynamics of transcriptional changes after CNS injury. Time-series data were generated from hippocampal CA1 neurons after transient forebrain ischemia. Approximately 100 CA1 cells were captured for each sample. RNA was amplified using TargetAmp (Epicentre Technologies) and analyzed using cDNA arrays as described by Kamme et al. (2003). The figure shows a manually selected subset of genes in a gray scale-coded cluster view. Each row corresponds to a gene. Data points in black represent down regulation (up to fourfold) with respect to the control group (in gray, first column), and white represents up regulation (up to fourfold). Time points after ischemia correspond to the columns seen from left to right: control, 2×1 h, 2×2 h, 2×4 h, 2×8 h, 2×16 h, 2×32 h, 2×64 h, 2×128 h, and 2×256 h. The gene-expression pattern is highly dynamic during the recovery phase after ischemic injury. The figure shows 151 out of a complete data set of 3115 genes.

microdissection and RNA amplification with the emerging high-throughput array platforms. Such an integrated system will enable the use of arrays in applications such as expression-based monitoring of drug effects *in vivo* (Gonzalez-Maeso et al., 2003). Along with improvements in data analysis, these methods promise a wealth of insight into several experimental paradigms relevant to the drug-discovery process.

REFERENCES

Ahram, M., Best, C.J., Flaig, M.J., Gillespie, J.W., Leiva, I.M., Chuaqui, R.F., Zhou, G., Shu, H., Duray, P.H., Linehan, W.M., Raffeld, M., Ornstein, D.K., Zhao, Y., Petricoin, E.F., III, Emmert-Buck, M.R. (2002). Proteomic analysis of human prostate cancer. *Mol. Carcinog.* 33: 9–15.

Bohm, M., Wieland, I., Schutze, K., Rubben, H. (1997). Microbeam MOMeNT: non-contact laser microdissection of membrane-mounted native tissue. *Am. J. Pathol.* 151: 63–67.

Bonaventure, P., Guo, H., Tian, B., Liu, X., Bittner, A., Roland, B., Salunga, R., Ma, X.J., Kamme, F., Meurers, B., Bakker, M., Jurzak, M., Leysen, J.E., Erlander, M.G. (2002). Nuclei and subnuclei gene expression profiling in mammalian brain. *Brain Res.* 943: 38–47.

Brady, G., Barbara, M., Iscove, N.N. (1990). Representative in vitro cDNA amplification from individual hematopoetic cells and colonies. *Methods Mol. Cell. Biol.* 2: 17–25.

Burbach, G.J., Dehn, D., Nagel, B., Del Turco, D., Deller, T. (2004). Laser microdissection of immunolabeled astrocytes allows quantification of astrocytic gene expression. *J. Neurosci. Methods* 138: 141–148.

Burgemeister, R., Gangnus, R., Haar, B., Schutze, K., Sauer, U. (2003). High quality RNA retrieved from samples obtained by using LMPC (laser microdissection and pressure catapulting) technology. *Pathol. Res. Pract.* 199: 431–436.

de la Fuente, A., Brazhnik, P., Mendes, P. (2002). Linking the genes: inferring quantitative gene networks from microarray data. *Trends Genet.* 18: 395–398.

Emmert-Buck, M.R., Bonner, R.F., Smith, P.D., Chuaqui, R.F., Zhuang, Z., Goldstein, S.R., Weiss, R.A., Liotta, L.A. (1996). Laser capture microdissection. *Science* 274: 998–1001.

Feldman, A.L., Costouros, N.G., Wang, E., Qian, M., Marincola, F.M., Alexander, H.R., Libutti, S.K. (2002). Advantages of mRNA amplification for microarray analysis. *Biotechniques* 33: 906–914.

Georgiou, H.M., Rice, G.E., Baker, M.S. (2001). Proteomic analysis of human plasma: failure of centrifugal ultrafiltration to remove albumin and other high molecular weight proteins. *Proteomics* 1: 1503–1506.

Goff, L.A., Bowers, J., Schwalm, J., Howerton, K., Getts, R.C., Hart, R.P. (2004). Evaluation of sense-strand mRNA amplification by comparative quantitative PCR. *BMC Genomics* 5: 76.

Goldsworthy, S.M., Stockton, P.S., Trempus, C.S., Foley, J.F., Maronpot, R.R. (1999). Effects of fixation on RNA extraction and amplification from laser capture microdissected tissue. *Mol. Carcinog.* 25: 86–91.

Gomes, L.I., Silva, R.L., Stolf, B.S., Cristo, E.B., Hirata, R., Soares, F.A., Reis, L.F., Neves, E.J., Carvalho, A.F. (2003). Comparative analysis of amplified and nonamplified RNA for hybridization in cDNA microarray. *Anal. Biochem.* 321: 244–251.

Gonzalez-Maeso, J., Yuen, T., Ebersole, B.J., Wurmbach, E., Lira, A., Zhou, M., Weisstaub, N., Hen, R., Gingrich, J.A., Sealfon, S.C. (2003). Transcriptome fingerprints distinguish hallucinogenic and nonhallucinogenic 5-hydroxytryptamine 2A receptor agonist effects in mouse somatosensory cortex. *J. Neurosci.* 23: 8836–8843.

Hariharan, R. (2003). The analysis of microarray data. *Pharmacogenomics* 4: 477–497.

Hughes, T.R., Marton, M.J., Jones, A.R., Roberts, C.J., Stoughton, R., Armour, C.D., Bennett, H.A., Coffey, E., Dai, H., He, Y.D., Kidd, M.J., King, A.M., Meyer, M.R., Slade, D., Lum, P.Y., Stepaniants, S.B., Shoemaker, D.D., Gachotte, D., Chakraburtty, K., Simon, J., Bard, M., Friend, S.H. (2000). Functional discovery via a compendium of expression profiles. *Cell* 102: 109–126.

Ji, W., Zhou, W., Gregg, K., Lindpaintner, K., Davis, S. (2004). A method for gene expression analysis by oligonucleotide arrays from minute biological materials. *Anal. Biochem.* 331:329-339.

Kaminski, N., Friedman, N. (2002). Practical approaches to analyzing results of microarray experiments. *Am. J. Respir. Cell Mol. Biol.* 27: 125–132.

Kamme, F., Zhu, J., Luo, L., Yu, J., Tran, D.T., Meurers, B., Bittner, A., Westlund, K., Carlton, S., Wan, J. (2004). Single-cell laser-capture microdissection and RNA amplification. *Methods Mol. Med.* 99: 215–223.

Kamme, F., Salunga, R., Yu, J., Tran, D.T., Zhu, J., Luo, L., Bittner, A., Guo, H.Q., Miller, N., Wan, J., Erlander, M. (2003). Single-cell microarray analysis in hippocampus CA1: demonstration and validation of cellular heterogeneity. *J. Neurosci.* 23: 3607–3615.

Leung, Y.F., Cavalieri, D. (2003). Fundamentals of cDNA microarray data analysis. *Trends Genet.* 19: 649–659.

Li, J., Adams, L., Schwartz, S.M., Bumgarner, R.E. (2003). RNA amplification, fidelity and reproducibility of expression profiling. *C. R. Biol.* 326: 1021–1030.

Lipshutz, R.J., Morris, D., Chee, M., Hubbell, E., Kozal, M.J., Shah, N., Shen, N., Yang, R., Fodor, S.P. (1995). Using oligonucleotide probe arrays to access genetic diversity. *Biotechniques* 19: 442–447.

Luo, L., Salunga, R.C., Guo, H., Bittner, A., Joy, K.C., Galindo, J.E., Xiao, H., Rogers, K.E., Wan, J.S., Jackson, M.R., Erlander, M.G. (1999). Gene expression profiles of laser-captured adjacent neuronal subtypes. *Nat. Med.* 5: 117–122.

Ma, X.J., Salunga, R., Tuggle, J.T., Gaudet, J., Enright, E., McQuary, P., Payette, T., Pistone, M., Stecker, K., Zhang, B.M., Zhou, Y.X., Varnholt, H., Smith, B., Gadd, M., Chatfield, E., Kessler, J., Baer, T.M., Erlander, M.G., Sgroi, D.C. (2003). Gene expression profiles of human breast cancer progression. *Proc. Natl. Acad. Sci. USA* 100: 5974–5979.

Moll, P.R., Duschl, J., Richter, K. (2004). Optimized RNA amplification using T7-RNA-polymerase based in vitro transcription. *Anal. Biochem.* 334: 164–174.

Mootha, V.K., Lindgren, C.M., Eriksson, K.F., Subramanian, A., Sihag, S., Lehar, J., Puig-server, P., Carlsson, E., Ridderstrale, M., Laurila, E., Houstis, N., Daly, M.J., Patter-son, N., Mesirov, J.P., Golub, T.R., Tamayo, P., Spiegelman, B., Lander, E.S., Hirschhorn, J.N., Altshuler, D., Groop, L.C. (2003). PGC-1alpha-responsive genes involved in oxidative phosphorylation are coordinately downregulated in human diabetes. *Nat. Genet.* 34: 267–273.

Mutsuga, N., Shahar, T., Verbalis, J.G., Brownstein, M.J., Xiang, C.C., Bonner, R.F., Gainer, H. (2004). Selective gene expression in magnocellular neurons in rat supraoptic nucleus. *J. Neurosci.* 24: 7174–7185.

Nishidate, T., Katagiri, T., Lin, M.L., Mano, Y., Miki, Y., Kasumi, F., Yoshimoto, M., Tsunoda, T., Hirata, K., Nakamura, Y. (2004). Genome-wide gene-expression profiles of breast-cancer cells purified with laser microbeam microdissection: identification of genes associated with progression and metastasis. *Int. J. Oncol.* 25: 797–819.

Ornstein, D.K., Gillespie, J.W., Paweletz, C.P., Duray, P.H., Herring, J., Vocke, C.D., Topalian, S.L., Bostwick, D.G., Linehan, W.M., Petricoin, E.F., III, Emmert-Buck, M.R. (2000). Proteomic analysis of laser capture microdissected human prostate cancer and in vitro prostate cell lines. *Electrophoresis* 21: 2235–2242.

Pabon, C., Modrusan, Z., Ruvolo, M.V., Coleman, I.M., Daniel, S., Yue, H., Arnold, L.J., Jr. (2001). Optimized T7 amplification system for microarray analysis. *Biotechniques* 31: 874–879.

Peterson, K.S., Huang, J.F., Zhu, J., D'Agati, V., Liu, X., Miller, N., Erlander, M.G., Jackson, M.R., Winchester, R.J. (2004). Characterization of heterogeneity in the molecular pathogenesis of lupus nephritis from transcriptional profiles of laser-captured glomeruli. *J. Clin. Invest.* 113: 1722–1733.

Phillips, J., Eberwine, J.H. (1996). Antisense RNA amplification: a linear amplification method for analyzing the mRNA population from single living cells. *Methods* 10: 283–288.

Polacek, D.C., Passerini, A.G., Shi, C., Francesco, N.M., Manduchi, E., Grant, G.R., Powell, S., Bischof, H., Winkler, H., Stoeckert, C.J., Jr., Davies, P.F. (2003). Fidelity and enhanced sensitivity of differential transcription profiles following linear amplification of nanogram amounts of endothelial mRNA. *Physiol. Genomics* 13: 147–156.

Rook, M.S., Delach, S.M., Deyneko, G., Worlock, A., Wolfe, J.L. (2004). Whole genome amplification of DNA from laser capture-microdissected tissue for high-throughput single nucleotide polymorphism and short tandem repeat genotyping. *Am. J. Pathol.* 164: 23–33.

Rudnicki, M., Eder, S., Schratzberger, G., Mayer, B., Meyer, T.W., Tonko, M., Mayer, G. (2004). Reliability of t7-based mRNA linear amplification validated by gene expression analysis of human kidney cells using cDNA microarrays. *Nephron. Exp. Nephrol.* 97: e86–95.

Schena, M., Shalon, D., Davis, R.W., Brown, P.O. (1995). Quantitative monitoring of gene expression patterns with a complementary DNA microarray. *Science* 270: 467–470.

Schneider, J., Buness, A., Huber, W., Volz, J., Kioschis, P., Hafner, M., Poustka, A., Sultmann, H. (2004). Systematic analysis of T7 RNA polymerase based in vitro linear RNA amplification for use in microarray experiments. *BMC Genomics* 5: 29.

Sherlock, G. (2001). Analysis of large-scale gene expression data. *Brief Bioinform.* 2: 350–362.

Spiess, A.N., Mueller, N., Ivell, R. (2003). Amplified RNA degradation in T7-amplification methods results in biased microarray hybridizations. *BMC Genomics* 4: 44.

Tavazoie, S., Hughes, J.D., Campbell, M.J., Cho, R.J., Church, G.M. (1999). Systematic determination of genetic network architecture. *Nat. Genet.* 22: 281–285.

Torres-Munoz, J.E., Van Waveren, C., Keegan, M.G., Bookman, R.J., Petito, C.K. (2004). Gene expression profiles in microdissected neurons from human hippocampal subregions. *Brain Res. Mol. Brain Res.* 127: 105–114.

Van Gelder, R.N., von Zastrow, M.E., Yool, A., Dement, W.C., Barchas, J.D., Eberwine, J.H. (1990). Amplified RNA synthesized from limited quantities of heterogeneous cDNA. *Proc. Natl. Acad. Sci. USA* 87: 1663–1667.

Wille, A., Zimmermann, P., Vranova, E., Furholz, A., Laule, O., Bleuler, S., Hennig, L., Prelic, A., von Rohr, P., Thiele, L., Zitzler, E., Gruissem, W., Buhlmann, P. (2004). Sparse graphical Gaussian modeling of the isoprenoid gene network in *Arabidopsis thaliana*. *Genome Biol.* 5: R92.

Xiang, C.C., Chen, M., Ma, L., Phan, Q.N., Inman, J.M., Kozhich, O.A., Brownstein, M.J. (2003). A new strategy to amplify degraded RNA from small tissue samples for microarray studies. *Nucleic Acids Res.* 31: e53.

Zhao, H., Hastie, T., Whitfield, M.L., Borresen-Dale, A.L., Jeffrey, S.S. (2002). Optimization and evaluation of T7 based RNA linear amplification protocols for cDNA microarray analysis. *BMC Genomics* 3: 31.

Zhu, J., Luo, L., Shi, T., Yu, J., Tran, D., Liu, X., Amaratunga, D., Bittner, A., Carmen, A., Wan, J., Chaplan, S., Kamme, F. (2004). Molecular cell-type definition in the rat dorsal root ganglion using single-cell gene expression profiling.

Index